T?
LEAN

A STRONG, ATHLETIC PHYSIQUE IN
JUST THREE HOURS PER WEEK

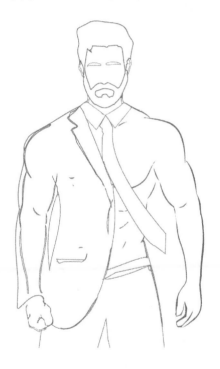

NEILL DAVID WATSON
WITH BIGGER BROTHER INSIGHT
FROM IAN ROSS WATSON

BIGGER BROTHER PUBLISHING
LONDON, UK

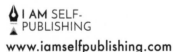 I AM SELF-
PUBLISHING

www.iamselfpublishing.com

DEDICATION

This book is dedicated to my wife, daughter, parents and my Bigger Brother, Ian, who have always been there for me. I also want to thank all the people throughout my life who have encouraged me and those people who have put me down. You have all been in some way my Bigger Brother helping me become a stronger and better individual with a desire to continually improve. For that, I am forever grateful.

NEILL DAVID WATSON

CONTENTS

DEFINITIONS

BIGGER BROTHER*

/BIH-GER BRUHTH-UR/

NOUN

Derived from the concept of "Standing on the shoulders of giants" – a person who has experience and knowledge they can share with you openly and impartially to help you avoid mistakes, improve and successfully reach your goals.

*This is a phrase and meaning created by the author based on the concept behind Bigger Brother. It's not in the dictionary or even the Urban Dictionary, although it should be and maybe one day it will be!

STANDING ON THE SHOULDERS OF GIANTS

The metaphor of dwarfs standing on the shoulders of giants (Latin: nanos gigantum humeris insidentes) expresses the meaning of "discovering truth by building on previous discoveries".

"If I have seen further, it is by standing on the shoulders of giants." **ISAAC NEWTON**

SYMMETRY

/SIM-I-TREE/

NOUN, PLURAL: SYMMETRIES.

1. The quality of being made up of exactly similar parts facing each other or around an axis.
2. Correct or pleasing proportion of the parts of a thing.

SYMMITARIAN**

/SIMI-TAIR-EE-UHN/

NOUN

A person who takes appropriate measures to develop their desired physique and mental state corresponding in form and arrangement, while balancing their lifestyle and goals.

**This is a word and meaning created by the author for this book. It's not in the dictionary or even the Urban Dictionary, although it should be and maybe one day it will be!

WHY SHOULD YOU READ THIS BOOK?

Firstly, and for the record, the author of this book was not a natural athlete and does not find training easy. Growing up, I was not particularly strong, fast or skilled at sport. At school, I was usually one of the last people to be picked for sports teams and I spent most of my teens warming the bench. I always had to work very hard at physical activity to improve or even compete with peers and would not be remembered by classmates for my sporting endeavours! This book is written on the back of 20 years of experience and knowledge gained through trial, error, lots of reading, learning, failure and success.

Secondly – as if you didn't know – your health is massively important!

If you want to live the longest and best life you can, staying healthy is a big part of that. The challenge is, you may also want to do well in your career, enjoy life and spend time with family and friends. Modern life doesn't tend to make it easy, particularly if you're an office executive that spends a lot of time indoors, sitting at a desk.

Studies have shown that success is often linked to good health and fitness.

PHYSICAL ACTIVITY IS ASSOCIATED WITH IMPROVED AFFECTIVE EXPERIENCE AND ENHANCED COGNITIVE PROCESSING.

THE NATIONAL CENTER FOR BIOTECHNOLOGY (NCBI)

STUDIES INDICATE THAT OUR MENTAL FIREPOWER IS DIRECTLY LINKED TO OUR PHYSICAL REGIMEN. AND NOWHERE ARE THE IMPLICATIONS MORE RELEVANT THAN TO OUR PERFORMANCE AT WORK.

HARVARD BUSINESS REVIEW, 2014

WITHOUT A DOUBT, THE HIGHER YOUR LEVEL OF FITNESS, THE GREATER THE CAPACITY YOU HAVE TO PERFORM YOUR JOB, AND THE GREATER CAPACITY YOU WILL HAVE TO DEAL WITH THE DEMANDS IN YOUR LIFE…

JACK GROPPEL, PHD, CO-AUTHOR OF *THE CORPORATE ATHLETE* (JOHN WILEY & SONS, 2000) AND CO-FOUNDER OF THE HUMAN PERFORMANCE INSTITUTE

Better fitness makes us better all-round performers. If you don't believe me, here's a quote I found online from my ultimate boss (at the time of writing, I work for Virgin Money):

I DEFINITELY CAN ACHIEVE TWICE AS MUCH BY KEEPING FIT.

RICHARD BRANSON, CO-FOUNDER OF THE VIRGIN GROUP

I have definitely found in my own life that, while staying fit can be a challenge and an effort to fit into daily life, making time for fitness, better eating and good sleep pays back tenfold in my productivity and career. It also teaches focus, consistency, helps to reduce stress, avoid sickness and problematic health issues, like back problems, pains and strains. It's worth noting that staying fit and healthy doesn't mean giving up on all the good things in life. I still enjoy delicious food (including burgers) and a beer or three. Actually, staying in shape allows me to indulge within reason, with limited impact on my health and fitness.

This book is for busy people who struggle to find time for fitness and want to balance work, life and health, minimising the time required to keep fit and maximising the benefits with a challenging schedule.

It will show you how, with the right focused effort, you can stay lean and fit in as little as three hours per week. I believe following the philosophy in this book, with the right balance in life, can make you fitter, healthier stronger and better – not just physically, but also mentally.

This is the Symmitarian Way.

WHO THIS BOOK IS FOR

(And Who It's Not For)

While this book includes and imparts information, knowledge, techniques and principles of professional fitness that can be used in, or lead to, building a physique fit for entry in a bodybuilding competition or a career in fitness modelling, it is not written specifically for people looking to develop this kind of professional career. This book is written for people who want to create and manage a fit, strong, muscular, lean, natural body at their own desired level – fitting it into their lives without having everything revolve around training and dieting.

Why? Because the reality is, even if you are genetically gifted, looking like a sub-10% body fat fitness model/bodybuilder usually requires a lot more time in the gym than most people (who are not doing it for their career) have time for, plus very strict dieting and possibly even some steroid use. If you need proof, just go online and search images for "off-season bodybuilders", "Arnold Schwarzenegger body" (to see how it varied through his 20s, 30s and 40s), or pictures of actor's beach bodies and compare them to how they look on screen. That's not to say there isn't work and effort involved and you can't maintain a great physique.

However, it doesn't have to rule your life and it's about finding a balance that feels good for you, not a secret pill or potion.

So, this book is for busy people who want to find and keep motivation and do the right things to see regular results in the development – and ultimately, maintenance – of a body they desire within a balanced lifestyle. Not to mention, still enjoy some cheeky treats without destroying progress. When considering what this book should be, here are some points that were noted down:

☑ Office executives, entrepreneurs and career-focused individuals who work above average hours and find it hard to get time in their schedules, but still want to be muscular, lean, and athletic.

☑ People with busy schedules who have to keep their exercise sessions and training to a minimum, but still want to maximise results.

☑ People who have let their fitness slip and want to get back into a regular, effective routine and return to good fitness.

☑ People who have thought about the benefits of weight training but aren't sure where to start or haven't gone to the gym for whatever reason.

☑ People who go to the gym but are not seeing the results they want.

☑ People who want to build muscle without drugs.

☑ Dads who want to stay fit to keep up with their kids.

☑ People who want to feel better, reduce stress and sleep better.

NOTE: WHILE THIS BOOK COULD BE USEFUL TO A WIDE VARIETY OF PEOPLE AND THE TECHNIQUES DESCRIBED ARE SUITABLE FOR MOST INDIVIDUALS LOOKING TO IMPROVE FITNESS, IT MAY PARTICULARLY APPEAL AND BE USEFUL TO MEN BETWEEN THE AGES OF 28 AND 55.

This book is designed for people who want to develop and maintain a solid, athletic, balanced, strong physique without it taking over their life, as well as wishing to avoid traps such as incorrect training and nutrition based on body attributes, not getting the results they want, plateaus, and loss of motivation. It's based on my own journey back to fitness and particularly written for people who are not "body professionals" (such as athletes or fitness models) who want to fit their fitness objectives around their life. By providing simple techniques, cutting through the bull$h*t and writing in layman's terms, this book will help get you on a long-term success track with training so you can (with the right attitude and effort):

☑   Avoid any fears and apprehension you may have about the gym and weight training (or getting back into it).

☑   Minimise fitness time but maximise results.

☑   Manage your own expectations.

☑   Stay motivated through the right techniques that deliver results for your natural body type.

☑   Take major steps to gaining a lean, athletic, strong physique.

☑   Start reaching your fitness goals with as little as three hours training per week.

☑   Improve sleep and reduce stress.

☑   Prepare to take on (or improve ability in) events like Tough Mudder, Spartan Race, Rat Race, etc...

WHY DID I WRITE THIS BOOK?

The Biggest Mistake Of My Life

That's right, one of the key reasons I wrote this book is because I made one of the biggest mistakes of my life in my late 20s. I stopped resistance training!! It didn't happen overnight, but gradually over about five years, and when I reached about 28 I stopped training and exercising completely!

Why did I let this happen?

I let my work take over and forgot some of the important things that weight training had taught me. I was working long hours, not sleeping well, partying and drinking in my free time and perhaps allowing stress to get the better of me. All that, hand in hand with the dregs from the bout of glandular fever I had at 20, caused recurring problems – and I let my health slip. I forgot, or chose to ignore, the benefits of health over other things in life, not to mention the great feeling that being fit and strong to the core gives you. I also forgot how powerful it can be, how it makes you more focused, efficient, helps you escape and helps you be better overall.

It wasn't until I was 32, a few days after my daughter was born, that I stood on the scales and couldn't believe the number I saw – 98kg (216lbs). As a guy who'd weighed

67kg (148lbs) 14 years earlier, and been a lean, muscular 88kg (194lbs) 6-7 years back, this was a shock. Not particularly because of the 10kg (22lbs) increase in weight, but because it dawned on me that my body composition had changed dramatically, and the reality was at least 20kg (44lbs) of that was now useless slush!!

It took a health issue after that for me to realise I had to force change. The challenge was also that the health issue made it trickier to lift weights (the doctor even suggested it would be worth trying to avoid lifting heavy weights to see if this would help). While I wouldn't condone ignoring your doctor's advice, I did some more research and decided I knew my body from the years of training I'd done before, and I knew if I ate better, cut down on the alcohol and built my body back the right way it would improve. I didn't leap into it, but started building from the ground up, step by step.

At first it was hard and there were quite a few setbacks, but I cut my fat down, increased muscle and took my training to a new level. That included increasing my one rep max on the deadlift from 80kg (176lbs) to 158kg (348lbs) and then up to 180kg (396lbs). I've never been a guy who wanted to be huge (particularly as it's not that useful in my efforts to learn to surf!), so a lean, strong weight of around 86-89kg (191-197lbs) works well for me. Below captures my initial body composition transition doing only three hours a week over eight (nearly nine) weeks - from being overweight and high body fat to my first phase of The Lean Exec:

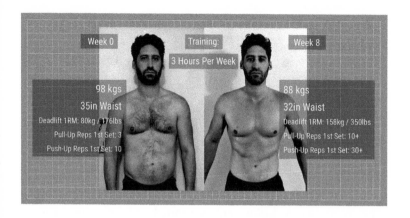

Week 0 — Training: 3 Hours Per Week — Week 8

Week 0	Week 8
98 kgs	88 kgs
35in Waist	32in Waist
Deadlift 1RM: 80kg / 176lbs	Deadlift 1RM: 158kg / 350lbs
Pull-Up Reps 1st Set: 3	Pull-Up Reps 1st Set: 10+
Push-Up Reps 1st Set: 10	Push-Up Reps 1st Set: 30+

NOTE: THESE IMAGES ARE COMPLETELY UNPREPARED SHOTS TAKEN WITH A SMARTPHONE CAMERA. NO SPECIFIC CUTTING DIET, NO TAN, ETC., JUST SENSIBLE EATING AND THREE HOURS' INTENSE TRAINING PER WEEK OVER THE EIGHT-WEEK PERIOD. I DRANK ALCOHOL, ALTHOUGH I CUT THIS DOWN TO NO MORE THAN SIX PINTS OF BEER PER WEEK. I ALSO STUCK TO QUALITY PALE ALES OR GUINNESS, WHERE THE ALCOHOL VOLUME WAS UNDER FIVE PER CENT. IN PRINCIPLE, YOU COULD TRAIN MORE AND BE MORE SPECIFIC WITH YOUR DIET TO POTENTIALLY ACHIEVE A LOWER BODY FAT PERCENTAGE, GREATER MUSCLE GAIN, INCREASED FITNESS, ETC. HOWEVER, I WANTED TO SHOW THE TECHNIQUES AND PRINCIPLES OF THE LEAN EXEC WORKED BASED ON MINIMAL ADJUSTMENTS WITH THREE HOURS' TRAINING PER WEEK, NOT DRAMATIC DIETS AND ENDLESS HOURS OF EXERCISE TIME.

AUTHOR STATS AT THE TIME OF WRITING THIS BOOK

Towards the end of writing this book, I tested for strength and strength endurance across some core exercises.

I used standards for males aged between 24–39, available online via sources such as Gym Jones, Bodybuilding.com, LiveStrong.com and StrengthLevel.com.

At age 40, commuting, working an average of 60–70 hours per week, balancing personal/family life and training, typically, three to five hours per week, I could hit high levels in the majority of the core resistance exercises.

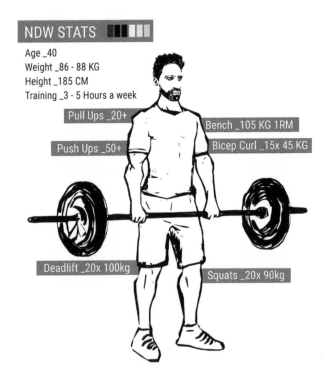

NDW STATS

Age _40
Weight _86 - 88 KG
Height _185 CM
Training _3 - 5 Hours a week

Pull Ups _20+

Bench _105 KG 1RM

Push Ups _50+

Bicep Curl _15x 45 KG

Deadlift _20x 100kg

Squats _20x 90kg

Move	Body Weight @ Test (KG)	Weight Lifted (KG)	No. of Reps (Tested)	1RM (kg) Tested	1RM (kg) Un-Tested (Based on 1REP Max calc)	Multiple of Body Weight (Tested)	Strength Endurance Standard*	Strength / Power Standard*	Level*
Back Squat	89	90	20	140	172	157%	20x @ Body Weight*	2x Body Weight male	Inter-Advanced
Deadlift	89	100	20	190	190	213%	25x @ 225lbs (102 KG)	2.5x Body Weight	Inter-Advanced
Bench Press	88	100	2	105	n/a	119%	n/a	1.5x Body Weight	Inter-Advanced
Barbell Curl (EZ)	88	45	15	n/a	73	83%	n/a	72kg = Advanced	Advanced
Pull-Ups (No Kips!)	87	Body	20	n/a	n/a	n/a	15x	n/a	Advanced
Push-Ups	87	Body	50	n/a	n/a	n/a	50x	n/a	Advanced
Plank	87	Body	2 Min+	2:30 - 3:00	n/a	n/a	2 Min	n/a	Advanced

*Sources: Gym Jones / Bodybuilding.com / StrengthLevel.com / LiveStrong.com

A WORD ON MOTIVATION

Motivation can be a very personal thing. I have found throughout my life that different things have motivated me to move and ultimately some things don't interest me enough to make me care. However, one philosophy I have that is rooted in Bigger Brother thinking is, if you care enough to complain or be bothered by something (which I'm guessing you are if you're reading this book?!), it can be channelled into motivation to change the situation.

When I first started weight training in my late teens, I was motivated by the fact that I wasn't particularly great at sports. I spent most of my time in the basketball team at senior school warming the bench. While I wasn't the weakest kid around and had no desire to be a huge bodybuilder, I was very thin, and I wanted to have a more athletic, muscular physique to boost my confidence (as well as appeal to the girls!). This is what initially drove me, but over time it was the positive feeling of being fitter and stronger that ultimately kept me going back to the gym.

Later in life, in my early 30s, when I was in the worst shape I had ever been in, the motivators that got me started again were quite different. I had made one of the biggest mistakes of my life by stopping training. I was unfit (to the point of being out of breath walking up a few stairs), unhealthy, overweight, stressed, suffering all sorts of ailments due to my condition and in need of a dramatic change. This time I was driven by a desire to feel better, to be healthier and, in particular, to be a healthy dad who could carry his daughter and keep up with her boundless energy. I didn't want to be one of those classic generalisations of being a dad with a pot belly, or – worst case scenario – die of something due to ill health. Of course, there are some things that you just can't control, but I figure I can do the best to stack the cards in my favour and hopefully I will have a long life. These things still drive me now to keep going, along with the positive feeling that comes with being fitter and stronger.

Beyond channelling negative gripes into positive motivation and drive, a good approach to failure is key. You have to get over that fear that you might fail. As clichéd as it might sound, failure is often a building block of success (for all bar a few lucky and unique examples who manage to avoid the experience). In addition, perhaps there is nowhere that the benefits of failure are more important or clear-cut than in exercise and resistance training.

In order to get stronger, better, faster, you must push forward to failure. The progress is in the failure of the muscles and their recovery. Our bodies are designed to adapt to failure and improve. I have also found that the understanding and appreciation of this failure through training has benefited me in all aspects of life. Obviously, you should not try to fail, but putting intense effort into succeeding and then failing can help you advance and the learnings from failure are often far more insightful than the successes they eventually lead to.

When I wrote the first draft of this section I found myself writing a lot of the usual bumf about motivation, like "what doesn't kill you makes you stronger", "once you can control your mind, you can control your body", "no pain, no gain" and so on. While some of the usual clichés have some truth in them, Bigger Brother does try to do things a little bit differently. So, here it is. The reality is, for most people, taking time out to go and train can be a pain in the a$$. Being conscious of what you eat and when can be annoying sometimes, and even downright awkward when you have a busy day. It's pretty normal to have days when it's really hard to get out of bed and face the world, let alone go to train.

When I went through my seven-year period of limited exercise, I was working long hours, drinking too much, not sleeping enough, feeling pretty yuck and regularly feeling ill and getting all sorts of niggles and ailments that I'd never had before. I think the ultimate realisation point for me was when I hurt my back and wasn't able to go to work for a few weeks. It was at that point I truly realised the mistake I had made. It took nearly six months for my back to totally recover, but with careful and consistent training it did recover to be far stronger than it's ever been. Within a year or so I could squat 135kg (297lbs), 10 rep sets with over 100kg (220lbs) and deadlift over 200% of my body weight which, at the time, was 88-90kg (198lbs). These numbers don't break any records, but they are significant and solid in the context of my goals.

The reality is, training can hit your body hard when you're doing it right; it can even feel uncomfortable at times and a bit like it's getting in the way of life. However, it's far better than the alternative. If you're training safely and correctly, although you might get soreness and niggles, your stronger body can fend off real issues that are damaging to you. Research shows that maintaining muscle also slows down the aging process. In addition, resistance training strengthens your bones and organs, not just your muscles. Plus, as you may have heard before, exercise releases endorphins that are positive and stress-relieving. The soreness of worked muscles can feel empowering, your body can feel cleaner and more capable, and it boosts confidence. Not to mention brain activity! The challenge is getting to the point where you start to feel these benefits – and this is where most people fall off the wagon.

As I will mention throughout this book, in principle, getting fit and optimising your body composition (note: I'm not referring to weight exclusively!) can be done at the same rate as your body gets out of shape. If you don't believe me, have a look at the workouts of Hollywood actors for major roles, where they transform their bodies in short spaces of time. Examples include the cast of 300, and recent superhero actors, including Henry Cavill and Ben Affleck. Of course, I hear you shout, "Don't they have experienced professionals managing every aspect of their time, nutrition and training?" Well, they do, but it doesn't mean you can't adapt a reasonable version of this that works within your lifestyle and financial reach. The important thing is not to set your expectations too high and align them with unrealistic goals. You have to adapt a pace and time frame that is realistic within your life and build it up over time. This is the route to longer term success.

Unfortunately, the world we live in means that it's much easier to slip into bad habits than to apply the small changes and effort needed to maintain fitness and health. It's hard to fight the lazy devil on one shoulder when the angel on the other can't offer you an easy way out. To get around this you will need to apply some reframing, focusing on the benefits and thinking of health and fitness as less of a chore and more of a way of life.

Getting motivated to do this doesn't need to be the big challenge it is often made out to be. Building it up to be something that is hard and seeing it as a chore only makes it seem harder than it really has to be. The combination of some simple knowledge, and a bit of consistency and balance, can soon make it easier to make a fit, healthy lifestyle part of your everyday routine. In addition, so much of the media and so called "advice" out there promotes a quick fix. While change can be quick at times, it's important to balance expectation and build up at a speed that is right for you. As previously mentioned, training gets easier the more your body becomes trained. Actually, scratch that; "easier" is probably not the right word. Training should be hard, otherwise you are not really pushing for improvement and maximising the opportunity for benefit. The difference is that as your body becomes more trained, it handles the training better, the training feels more empowering, and even enjoyable, which helps you to be motivated. Training makes you feel good and, as you get into it, you even crave it, making it easier to maintain regular training.

A word of warning, though. Prior to getting to the point where you really understand your body and can read what it's telling you, you are in danger of giving up. While it's important to train intensely, overdoing it or over training can kill motivation and progress. Training intensely for your level within your capacity to recover is key, particularly at the start of the journey and before you have reached a reasonable maintenance mode.

Here are Bigger Brother's laws of motivation to get you started:

☑ Don't be afraid to start small. It doesn't matter how light the weight (or short the run) is, as long as it is right for you and your goals. Just be sure to get out there and focus on building.

☑ Plan to keep it short, because: A) 10 mins is better than 0; and, B) starting is the hardest part. Once you start, going for longer than 10 mins may happen naturally.

☑ Make it easier to go to exercise:

- Join a gym near to work or your home.

- Get it out of the way by training in the morning.

- Prepare your gym bag the night before.

- Jog, cycle or skate to the gym. Not only will it help you warm up, it will make it easier once you get there. The hardest thing to do is start; once you're in motion, it's easier to continue.

☑ Make it easier to exercise:

- Don't go to the gym having not eaten for more than three hours. Having some good quality food one to two hours before training will ensure you have the right energy levels to train intensely. Bigger Brother likes a light banana protein shake with at least 20 grams of protein, plus 40 grams of quality Scottish porridge oats, about one to two hours before training.

- Have a coffee or two, one hour before training. If you like espresso, then that's ideal, as it keeps the calories low. Bigger Brother doesn't think there is any issue with a bit of milk (unless you're allergic to it, of course), but stick to skimmed milk (minimal fat) and keep it under 50ml a cup until you are in maintenance mode and have a bit more flexibility. If you don't like coffee or can't have it for any reason, then some caffeine supplements or drinks may work; just ensure you read the labels to be certain it's quality and not full of fat, sugar or calories. Bigger Brother prefers coffee as it's natural and finds it works great!

- Ensure the pre-workout food has settled before you train. Training when your stomach still feels full can be uncomfortable.

- Warm up! Start with simple stretching, a jog or an easier weight to get the blood flowing.

☑ If you can't get motivated to trek to the gym, do some body weight exercise at home.

☑ Find a friend to train with and help motivate each other. If you're a loyal friend, setting a time to meet at the gym will ensure you can't just sack it off because you don't feel like it. Also, you can motivate each other with a bit of friendly competition banter!

☑ Hang out with more people who have fit and healthy lifestyles and eating habits; this will naturally rub off on you.

☑ If you don't like running, swimming or cycling, find something else you enjoy – ideally something you did while growing up. Skate, surf, snowboard, play football, rugby, basketball, or whatever appeals to you to get your fitness up. If you enjoy doing a sport it may help encourage you to exercise more, as playing is fun.

☑ Try reading inspiring stories about people who have overcome challenges.

☑ It's clichéd but think positively and concentrate on the benefits and the goal you want to reach, but do make sure the goal is broken down into small steps, so you can see the progress developing over time.

☑ Make sure you're as comfortable as you can be:

- Forget style and look, get yourself some comfortable training gear.

- Have a warm bath after training. You can also try a cold or ice bath, which is popular amongst athletes aiming to reduce the body stresses of a hard workout.

THE IDEA IS THAT IMMERSING THE BODY IN FREEZING COLD WATER SPEEDS UP RECOVERY AFTER EXERCISE BY REDUCING TEMPERATURE, BLOOD FLOW AND INFLAMMATION IN TISSUES OF THE MUSCLES.

SOURCE: BBC.CO.UK

- If you are sore from previous training, try things like Deep Heat and Deep Freeze on the sore areas to help relieve discomfort.

- Ensure you are eating both the correct macro-nutrients and micronutrients to support your body's needs.

- Try some supplements that help with joint pain and support recovery. Don't go mad, as lots of supplements just mean an expensive number one, but some supplements are known to be helpful. For more on Supplements, go to:

  BIT.LY/TLE-SUPP

- Get more sleep. Scientists still don't fully understand why we have to sleep or how much exactly we really need, but it's recognised that it benefits recovery and performance. How much sleep you need seems to depend on genetics, but many athletes swear sleep is key to their ability to train and perform at the highest levels. In any case, it's worth trying to have some more sleep and see how it impacts your recovery and performance in daily life, not just in the gym, but mentally too. Here are some quotes from athletes about their sleep which can be easily found by searching online:

SLEEP IS EXTREMELY IMPORTANT TO ME – I NEED TO REST AND RECOVER IN ORDER FOR THE TRAINING I DO TO BE ABSORBED BY MY BODY.

USAIN BOLT

IF I DON'T SLEEP 11 TO 12 HOURS A DAY, IT'S NOT RIGHT.

ROGER FEDERER

EAT, SLEEP, AND SWIM, THAT'S ALL I CAN DO.

MICHAEL PHELPS

As with anything in life, getting started is often the hardest part. The second hardest part is being realistic with your goals. Unfortunately, it's rare that things happen overnight. There tends to be a hockey stick shaped growth curve, where things are slow and most difficult at the start, but then begin to grow more rapidly as momentum starts to build. It's not that you shouldn't aim high, ultimately, it's just that it's important to remember that things often take longer than expected and require more effort than expected to get going, so it's key to be realistic with those expectations. Otherwise, you risk continually missing the small targets that will get you to that ultimate goal. If you're realistic and attack small chunks at a time, you will start to see small incremental results which will help to keep you motivated.

TRAINING TO BE THE LEAN EXEC

Not everyone wants to be a professional body athlete, like a bodybuilder or fitness model, and to be that takes substantial dedication to training and nutrition – although the comments from admirers on the beach may be enough incentive for some to achieve similar levels. As mentioned throughout the book, the tools, techniques and knowledge within can be applied at a range of levels to achieve desired results, but the main focus is on helping people find the balance they want to achieve with fitness and health, alongside their everyday life.

It's Bigger Brother's belief that health is one area where, for most people, what you do – with consideration given to your genetics – can directly correspond to the results. In principle, nobody else's actions need have any impact on your results. That's something that can't be said for many things in life. If you consistently do the right things for *you*, 50% of the time, the output will be 50% of your potential. Similarly, if you get to know yourself and what works for you and do it consistently 60%, 70%, 80%, 90% of the time, your results will most likely match. If we were to say the average body was 50%–60%, then you only need an additional 5% or 10% to start having above average lean fitness.

Therefore, the formula might be portrayed as:

(CORRECT TRAINING FOR BODY + (APPROPRIATE NUTRITION + SUITABLE REST FOR TRAINING)) X 80% CONSISTENCY = 80% OF YOUR OPTIMAL HEALTH AND FITNESS

Now, this is not really scientific (or perhaps it's Bigger Bro Science ☺), but the concept is sound and rooted in experienced results. Whatever percentage of time you spend doing the right things will be equal to the percentage of the potential results you obtain. This, in particular, applies to food, but in principle, if you spend 80% of your time sitting on the sofa, at a desk, eating crap and doing no exercise, you'll most likely be overweight and unhealthy. If you spend 80% of your time applying healthy habits, then your body will reflect that, and that still leaves 20% of the time for some fun and indulgence (if you want it). What's interesting is that, as you get past 80% (or even 70%), you become less interested in doing what's in the remaining 20%, because the 80% feels so good! So, it becomes less of a chore and more a way of life.

To get there is a process and does require effort, but the following chapters of this book are designed to impart in-depth knowledge and help you progress to your desired level faster. Maximising efficiency and benefit so you can see results sooner will motivate you to continue. It's the author's, and Bigger Brother's, aim for this to be the only book you need to get you from your current status to a position where you can manage and get the benefits of ongoing fitness without it taking over your life. However, we would encourage you to continue reading and widening your knowledge, as it will only help in your quest to become a Symmitarian (definition at the start of this book).

GET REAL, DUDE!

Exercise and training isn't meant to be easy, no matter what genetics you were born with. Yes, it's true that some people are more naturally gifted in lean muscle building and fitness, but even they have to put in the hours. Arnold Schwarzenegger spent five hours a day, six days a week, training with ruthless discipline, and followed a strict diet regime for years to build that famous physique. Apparently, when his legs were his weak points, he hammered them with thousands of pounds of weights, three times a week. So, to look/be strong, lean and muscular, you need to move some weight around, in more ways than one.

For most of us, five hours a day in the gym isn't a realistic target and we're not all training for Mr. Olympia, the Olympic Games, or the next comic book superhero movie. Luckily, with the right approach for your body type, some simple thought about your diet and some reasonable effort, you can improve your body significantly, whether it's for strength, fitness, aesthetics or all three.

If you are new to training or hold any anxiety about the gym – i.e. being around stronger, leaner, more athletic people – don't worry. If you feel self-conscious about your body, don't. Most gyms are full of a mix of people in varying shape and everyone there had a first day in the gym. No one is going to laugh at you for showing up and making some effort, and if they do, they're not worth thinking about. It's worth remembering that even the most confident and advanced guys in your gym will remember what it was like when they started. Plus, everyone has their own strengths and weak points, versus someone else's.

The great thing is, just by reading this book, you'll already know more than a good portion of average gym-goers, even some of the ones whose bodies make them look like they know what they're doing (and perhaps even some of the PTs!). Once you've read this you can start on the right path and avoid looking like a clumsy gym zombie, wandering around hoping what you are doing will get you fit and strong.

THE 10 COMMANDMENTS OF TRAINING

ADAPTED FROM THE 10 COMMANDMENTS OF GYM TRAINING, BY MY BIGGER BROTHER, IAN ROSS WATSON.

I. THE BIG(GER) SECRET IS... THERE IS NO SECRET!!

People only hear what they want to hear. It's common sense. It's logical. If you put effort into the right exercise and nutrition, you will get results. Everyone wants to hear, "Go out and lift a pencil for 30 seconds, then eat a kebab and a bag of chips, finish your workout by washing it all down with five pints of beer, then take a break – you deserve it!"

No one wants to hear, "Exercise intensely in line with your desired goals, eat nutritious food in appropriate quantities related to your body's demands, drink sufficient amounts of water. Select foods which are fibrous, complex, unrefined, provide sufficient protein, give you essential amino acids, are not processed, and are not excessively high in saturated fat, and don't overeat carbohydrates."

Be smart; don't listen to drivel! And, before you ask, "How do I know this is not drivel?" Well, the truth is, you don't, which is exactly the point. Use common sense. If it makes sense, that's because the methods are based on accurate information, not gossip magazine and news article speculation, generic fads, or fringe studies carried out on micro-samples of people by a supplement manufacturer wishing you to buy their product, but basic principles that work.

II. IF YOU WANT TO LOOK AND FEEL GOOD, YOU MUST EXERCISE

You often hear people exclaiming how proud they are that they have just lost five kilograms by starving themselves and doing no exercise. Great, they just lost five kilograms, but five kilograms of what?

They might have lost four kilos of muscle and only one kilo of fat, in which case their body fat has stayed pretty much the same and they've sacrificed four kilos of their fat-burning powerhouse – muscle!

When people diet in this fashion, their body, in fact, loses the majority of its weight in the form of fat-free mass (FFM) and not fat mass (FM). The latter is what you should aim to lose. Many people seem to disregard the composition of their weight loss and instead go for measuring the pure poundage. Not only is the majority of the weight lost in this fashion FFM, but the participant in this kind of diet has also slowed their metabolism down considerably due to this loss. This ensures that when a normal diet is resumed, their body has, in fact, become less adept at coping with their caloric intake. That means more calories are stored as fat and less fat is burned.

To prevent this happening, you must exercise and eat to improve your muscle-to-fat ratio. Doing this correctly makes your body more adept at burning fat, because it raises your metabolism, giving your body a higher threshold for fat usage. This is great, because it means that you will burn more fat even when doing absolutely nothing! Your metabolism is raised because effective training promotes protein synthesis which, combined with an appropriate diet, enables you to gain more FFM, making you even better at burning fat while doing nothing. This makes your body burn more fat every hour of the day, and more still, when exercising.

Remember, it is ultimately about losing "fat", not about losing "weight" and, equally, it's about increasing "lean (muscle) mass", not increasing "weight". The mirror can often be a much better benchmark for progress than a set of scales.

III. WE ARE ALL HUMAN

This is an important rule, as the reality is, even the pros let things slip at some point in their lives, even (especially) Bigger Brother! The bad diet period, a drop in exercise frequency, reduced effort, and/or the binge drinking session – all are part of being human.

The key thing is, if you are guilty, don't dismiss it and reward yourself. Don't kid yourself that what you are doing is good for you. Here's an example:

How often have you heard someone say, "Ooh! I'll eat this chocolate bar, because cocoa is good for you, you know? And it gives you loads of energy, which is really important," or, "Tomato ketchup is a good source of vitamins, tomatoes can help prevent prostate cancer," or how about, "Mayonnaise must be good for you, it's made from egg whites, and they're good for you, aren't they?"

The point is, eat the chocolate bar, smother your food in ketchup until your chips are positively swimming in it, don't put the recommended tablespoon of mayo on your sandwich, slather it in the stuff if you want. Just don't kid yourself it's doing you any good! Again, common sense is paramount. A miniscule proportion of less healthy food may be doing you some good, but these are far outweighed by the negative effects. Sure, tomato ketchup is made from tomatoes, but it often contains piles of refined sugar in every tablespoon. A bit of chocolate won't do you any harm, it might put you in a positive frame of mind, but the block of butter and excessive sugar that went into making that chocolate won't do you any favours.

That's not to say you can't embrace it at times and enjoy the less healthy things in life. One of the things that differs in the Bigger Brother methodology from some other training and diet methods is a realisation that you can balance your fitness with regular treats, allowing you to embrace the demons occasionally, alongside the longer periods when you need to keep things under control.

IV. YOUR DIET MUST BE APPROPRIATE FOR THE DEMANDS YOU ARE PLACING ON YOUR BODY

We often hear people brag that they worked out or ran for three hours and haven't eaten anything. These people don't have a clue! Let them go on bragging about their training and diet regimen – you know the truth (or at least you will, after reading this book!).

It's always amazing to see how our wider society perpetuates the fallacy that raising your level of activity should automatically be coupled with eating less. Yes, exercise is very important, and it is good to be keen, but not when it becomes detrimental to your goals. In fact, not eating in line with your body's demands is called malnutrition. This seems like a word which is only associated with starving populations in developing nations, but people do it to themselves after workout sessions across the world. Either that, or they do a workout and then eat something unhealthy as a "reward"!

V. LESS CAN BE MORE & THE LAW OF DIMINISHING RETURNS

This is a concept most people really don't seem to be familiar with in gyms – anywhere! We have all been brought up to believe that in order to achieve things we must work hard at them and put in a lot of effort. While there is truth in that, it doesn't automatically mean an excessive demand on our time.

Longer time spent in the gym is not directly correlated to success. I guarantee you that you will make far more progress (and spend far less time in the gym) if you run as hard as you can repeatedly, in short bursts (intervals), over 20–30 minutes, than you will by jogging at a snail's pace for 45 minutes. This is because intensity can be more important than time. Please do not confuse what I am trying to say here. Effort does have a high correlation with results, but "effort", expressed in terms of time spent doing an activity, doesn't necessarily.

Numerous studies have shown that shorter (under one hour), more intense sessions, coupled with appropriate recuperation and nutrition, can deliver better results than either long, low intensity or over-extended training sessions that result in over-training the body. What is important is that you can achieve more in the first 30 minutes of a solid workout, than in the remaining two and a half hours of a three-hour sloppy one!

VI. REST IS PARAMOUNT TO SUCCESS (EXERCISE WITHIN YOUR ABILITY TO RECUPERATE)

So, tonight you're heading out on the town! Good stuff, better head to the gym to make sure you look a bit better for the ladies/men, before you get "battered like a fish". Great workout! You reached new heights of physical exertion, time to get a shower and meet your friends. At 2am you return from your social expedition, head pounding after being pummelled by decibels from the nearby 100,000-watt speakers in the nightclub/bar, or your mate shouting in your ear. Not to mention the 10 pints/2 bottles of wine/12 tequila slammers reducing your chemical manhood (testosterone) to a fraction of its normal levels. It's no surprise you feel like absolute s**t, and all you want now is a nice soft pillow.

Despite the training the day before, your trip to the gym hasn't done you much good, either. Not only have you hammered your body into physical submission, but you also haven't rewarded yourself (or your body) for it by giving it some prolonged nutrition and recuperation. Not only did you get up at 6am yesterday morning, but you scurried around all day, hit the gym for some serious weight shifting and topped it off with an all-nighter.

After putting away copious amounts of calorie-laden alcohol, you bombarded your digestive system with some reconstituted "hoof" from your local eating house. This has resulted in you starting on the well-trodden path of growing saggy breasts, by not only exerting yourself beyond the point of your ability to recuperate, but also refusing to give your body the nutrition it requires. Alcohol is, without a doubt, a devil in disguise for multiple reasons and, while you can get away with some consumption within your target calories in a week, it is more than likely hindering very real progress, particularly when combined with little rest and poor nutrition.

If you want to drink and also train, it is possible to balance a fit physique and some alcoholic pleasure, but frequent excessive drinking is not recommended. Also, most people over 25 or who do not have an exceptionally fast metabolism will struggle to get a fitness model or competition body look without removing alcohol from their diet. There is no real "advice" for drinking and training, as you shouldn't really do it. However, if you do have a night out, make sure you eat very well on the days around it and save a few calories, without dropping macronutrients (more on macronutrients later in the book). Avoid being in a state of delayed onset muscle soreness (DOMS) from previous training, pace yourself, ensure you can get some additional rest the day after, and do some extra cardio a few days before and after the drinking, once rested and nourished.

VII. STOP EXERCISING YOUR "PINKY" AND WORK ON YOUR DEADLIFTS & SQUATS

Arrrgh! That was a yell of frustration. The next "dweeb" I see in the gym exercising his *wrist* with the latest move he got out of a muscle mag will be sent home!

While I'm trying to deadlift some serious poundage and achieve some real progress in my training, Sammo Skinny, in the corner over there with his nine-inch biceps, is looking at me as he does his wrist curls, wondering how he can get strong.

Slightly exaggerated, but the point is, until you have a basic athletic physique you will need to build some overall strength, so stick to the fundamentals. Compound movements first, isolation moves later. I'm not a beginner, but I certainly don't start my main workouts off with a bicep curl, and neither would the pros. Stick to the "meat and potatoes" exercises, they will do far more for your wrist strength than any wrist workout will.

A SPECIAL NOTE FOR MR (OR MS) WRIST STRAP SUPPORT: UN-LESS YOU'RE AN EXPERIENCED STRONGMAN OR BODYBUILDER AND REALLY KNOW WHAT YOU'RE DOING, IF YOU CAN'T LIFT IT WITHOUT WRIST STRAP SUPPORT, THEN DROP THE WEIGHT AND WORK ON LIFTING WELL WITHOUT SUPPORT, INCREASE THE WEIGHT, REPEAT OVER TIME. IF YOU ALWAYS USE WRIST SUPPORT, YOU'RE NOT PARTICULARLY HELPING YOUR WRISTS GET STRONGER.

VIII. MACHINES ARE FOR VARIETY, AFTER THE "BREAD AND BUTTER"

This is closely linked to Rule VII. Stop getting entwined in the cables, involved in the pec deck and intimate with the ab-isolator – ignore the sales spin on machines or exercise fads.

Truth be told – and people with certain health issues aside – in most cases, these are only really useful (there are exceptions) as supplementary pieces of equipment.

How did people get so developed in the days when they only had a barbell, rack and chin-up bar? Answer: They stuck to fundamental exercises that helped their physique develop in unison, because that was all the equipment would allow.

Bigger Brother is fully confident in stating that you could achieve an extremely muscular, desirable, symmetrical body using no more than a few movements – deadlift/bench press/squat/chin-up/barbell curls/shoulder (military) press/row. How can Bigger Brother be so sure? Well, because based on his autobiography, *Total Recall*, that's pretty much what Arnold Schwarzenegger did for the first few years, creating the foundation for his world-renowned physique. Then there's the legendary classic bodybuilder, Steve Reeves (if you don't know who Steve Reeves is, just do a quick search online).

Unfortunately, machines in gyms are not a like-for-like comparison with other technology advancements. While they are not bad, as such, they are not as effective as much of the basic free weight equipment. Quite often, in modern gyms, they take up most of the space and distract from the really useful equipment that should be the main event.

IX. YOUR BODY IS LIKE A CAR, BUT IT IS NOT A CAR

The analogy of comparing the body to a car is a useful one, because it is something most people will be familiar with.

In the same way that you fill a car with fuel, you fill your body with food (a lesson in fuel economies):

☑ If you fill your petrol car with vegetable oil, it will not start or will, at best, run poorly. Similarly, if you fill your body with inappropriate food, you will feel lethargic and demotivated.

☑ If you fill your car with good petrol that is highly refined, it will run at its best. Unlike a car, your body will not perform well if you feed it "good" tasting food that is highly refined. Instead, your body will perform best if you fill it with nutritious food that is less refined.

☑ The longer your car goes, the more fuel it requires. Like your car, the longer your body exercises for, the more food it needs.

☑ The faster your car accelerates, the less efficient it becomes. Like your car, the faster you accelerate, the less efficient you become. Unlike your car, your body becomes more efficient as time passes and you continue exercising and feeding it well.

In the same way that your car has gears, so too do the muscles in your body:

☑ The faster your car goes, the higher the gear that is required. The faster you go, the more involvement is required from the larger motor units controlling your muscle fibres.

☑ The faster your car goes, the sooner you need to refuel it. The faster you go, the sooner your body becomes tired and needs to rest.

☑ The slower and more consistent your car goes, the further your car will travel. The slower you go, the further your body can travel.

☑ The slower your car goes, the lower the gear it requires. The slower you go, the more your body can rely on your baseline oxygen energy systems.

In the same way you take care of a car, you must take care of your body:

If you "grind" the gears in your car too often, you will wreck the gearbox and have to replace it. If you carry out exercise movements incorrectly, you will create wear and tear on your ligaments and this will lead to injury. Unlike gearboxes, joints cannot be replaced (or at least, not quite as easily and not without challenges).

X. IN ORDER TO KNOW HOW TO EXERCISE EFFECTIVELY, YOU MUST HAVE TRAINED MUSCLE

Life is a bi**h, as they say, and exercise is no different. Unfortunately, in a chicken-and-egg kind of way, knowing how to exercise instinctively and effectively requires you to already have or have had trained muscle.

The "fitter" our muscles become, the more aware we become of them. Similarly, if we have had trained muscles before and let them slip, we will find it easier to regain the awareness and fitness (sometimes referred to as "muscle memory"). In this manner, it becomes easier for the highly trained individual to know whether their training is effective or not. Trained individuals develop a "feel" for what is working their muscles during exercise and, as a consequence, can train more effectively.

Well-developed muscles act like a negative feedback mechanism; they allow the exerciser to more accurately gauge the effect the workload is having upon particular muscles. This can, however, be easily overcome, by ensuring that the exerciser has adequate knowledge of technique and the demands they are placing upon the body and its resultant effects in terms of physiological adaptations. By employing an effective training programme, the beginner in resistance exercise can become increasingly aware of how their body is working in a short space of time.

STORY TIME: LEGEND OF THE SYMMITARIAN

Long ago, in a time long forgotten, there was a boy who dreamed of being a champion. He lived in a small village in ancient Europe. The homes of the village were built into the foot of a hill, in a clearing surrounded by thick evergreen trees. The terrain was rough, the weather unforgiving and the forests filled with danger, from great beasts to rival village warriors. The village was small, but it was the oldest village in the area. It had withstood countless storms and enemy attacks and the longstanding survival of its people was legendary for miles around.

The strength of the village lay in its balance, and the way teachings and methodologies passed down through generations. They did not have the strongest man – he could be found in the village of Endo – or the best endurance runner; he lived on the flatlands, in the village of Ecto.

However, overall, the village of Meso, in Symmitaria, had the most versatile and adept group of hunters, warriors, skilled craftsmen and knowledge-bearers in the land. The villagers of Meso were not all born with natural abilities; it was the knowledge passed through ancestry that gave them their skills and strengths.

The boy's father was one of the village's finest warriors, known for his combination of strength, speed and manoeuvrability. He had also risen up the ranks of the village community and was a respected member of the village knowledge-bearers. Even when he was extremely busy with his duties in the village, he would spend an hour per day lifting logs, doing pull-ups on trees, or running after his children. He always took time to sleep sufficiently and would eat multiple times during the day. The food was simple: small amounts of chicken and freshly grown vegetables. Like any of the village men, at times he would feast on exotic and delicious foods and drink ales, but for the most part he ate nutrient-dense foods and frequently encouraged his son to do the same.

One day, the small boy's father took him on a trading visit to the nearest villages. An hour or so before leaving, they ate a hearty breakfast of eggs and delicious oats, in preparation. They set out on the hour-long jog through tough, muddy terrain. The boy had started his warrior training, but still found it hard to keep up with his father, whose lean, muscled physique seemed to bounce over the earth and slide up and over any of the large obstacles with relative ease.

When they arrived at the first village, the boy's father handed him a piece of chicken, an apple and some fresh water. The boy raised a tired arm, took the food and quickly gobbled it up. His muscles ached and he was tired, but invigorated.

As they walked through the village, the boy saw a huge man with a large belly – he looked almost like a modern-day strongman. He was massive and heavy, seated in a large chair, eating what looked like enough food for a whole village. At that moment another villager looked up from his work on a half-finished stone and mud hut and called out to him, beckoning him over. The giant man put down his bowl and, using his thick arms, leveraged his enormous, heavy body up and onto his feet. As he walked over to his fellow villager it was as if the ground shook with each step. He was slow, but powerful.

As he reached his comrade, the boy saw a large cart filled with mud and stone, some of which was being used to build the hut. The giant man stepped forward towards the cart and, with relative ease, lifted the handles, then rolled the cart, along with its heavy contents, to the other side of the hut and set it down. The two villagers nodded at each other, then the hulking man returned to his chair, picked up his bowl and carried on eating.

The boy's father yelled over to him and the boy jogged on to catch up with his father. The boy had been amazed by the man's size and strength and as he walked further on through the village he noticed many of the villagers were bulky, large, and, he could imagine, strong, like the man he saw move the cart.

The boy and his father completed their trade with the chief tradesman in Endo and set out on the three-quarters of an hour journey to the village of Ecto, the last stop on their day trip. The journey to Ecto was across much flatter terrain, but father and son had to cross a wild rushing river on a thin double rope and paddle half a mile across the great lake. The boy worked hard to keep up with his father, making up for his lack of strength with his youthful endurance.

As they reached the village of Ecto, the boy saw a group of slender men with spears jogging into the village, carrying what looked like a dead deer. The boy's father explained that they were Ecto hunters returning from a three-day hunt across the plains. The men looked tiny compared to the men in his village, although despite their slim, stringy frames and almost malnourished look, they jogged with vigour, showing little sign of tiredness despite the multi-day marathon they had just completed. As the men passed by, the boy noticed one man reach into a small sack around his waist and pull out a handful of nuts and berries, then toss them into his mouth. He chomped as he ran. The boy's father went on to explain that these Ecto hunters were known for their endurance and would often run for days across the plains in search of prey to kill and bring back to feed the village.

The father and son finished their business in the village and hiked over the plains, great lake, up and down the hills back to their home in the village of Meso.

On their return, the boy was tired, but 20 minutes after he arrived he was sitting with his family eating a large portion of fish, sweet potatoes and fresh vegetables. The taste was fantastic, as he felt the benefit of the nourishment through his tired body. Later that evening, he ate a bowl of his favourite milk rice, a special recipe of the village that blended milk by-products with natural coconut flavoured essence and Theobroma cacao. The magnesium that was naturally found in the dish was also believed to help improve sleep.

The young Symmitarian wrapped himself up in his warm bed and listened to his bigger brother share experiences from his day's training. He knew that if he wanted to become a great warrior, like his father and bigger brother, he would need to learn as much as he could, and that the knowledge would help him to accelerate his progress. His muscles felt tired from the day, but he felt good as he nodded off into a restful sleep, happy that his body would begin to grow stronger over the coming days and weeks.

GET TO KNOW YOUR BODY

BODY ATTRIBUTES

Unfortunately, despite what people say, we are not all created equal – at least, not physically. Note, I am not referring to general human rights and equality, here. The reality is, our genetics vary and we naturally come in all different shapes and sizes (it's part of what makes life interesting!). In principle, this includes how naturally good our bodies are at gaining muscle, losing fat, running fast, long-distance racing, power, etc...

NOTE: THERE IS A REALLY INTERESTING DOCUMENTARY FROM CHANNEL 4 PRESENTED BY OLYMPIAN MICHAEL JOHNSON, CALLED *SURVIVAL OF THE FASTEST*, WHICH RAISES SOME INTERESTING AND PERHAPS CONTROVERSIAL POINTS ABOUT GENETICS AND ATHLETICISM.

Just think back to your schooldays. There are, of course, exceptions to the rule, but you can probably remember one person who was extremely thin, another who was muscular and athletic, and another who was overweight. Possibly you were one of those described, or a mix. I was tall and skinny, despite eating plenty of calories.

At this point it's worth highlighting the theory of somatotypes. Somatotypes is a taxonomy that was developed in the 1940s that put people into different categories, based on the extent to which their bodily physique, particularly their skeletal frame, conforms to a basic type, e.g. thin, muscular, dense.

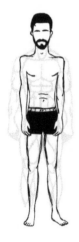 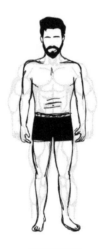 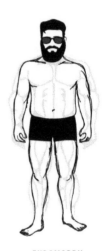

ECTOMORPH
NATURALLY SLIM BUILD
SMALL SKELETAL FRAME

MESOMORPH
NATURALLY ATHLETIC BUILD
MEDIUM SKELETAL FRAME

ENDOMORPH
NATURALLY HEAVY BUILD
LARGE SKELETAL FRAME

Essentially, somatotypes refer to the underlying physique which, in principle, is not easily changed by diet or training. There is a lot of discussion and many different views about how real or useful somatotypes are in determining your "potential". I won't go into it in detail here, as a quick Internet search can give you that information. However, Bigger Brother believes, while you shouldn't take somatotypes too literally, common-science (see what I did there) and experience tells us it's worth understanding your body's strengths and weaknesses better, to optimise your progress.

The reality is, whatever you believe, most people are a mix of body types, although "pre-training" seem to lean closer to one of the somatotype groups – Ectomorph, Mesomorph and Endomorph. The good news is you can evolve your body and with a good understanding of your body response can maximise your training and nutrition to your goals and reaching the success you're looking for.

The theory behind somatotypes is that each body type has its advantages and disadvantages when it comes to the quest to sculpt a body ideal, although it is generally easier for a mesomorph to gain lean muscle mass (that doesn't necessarily mean they don't have to work hard too!). Ultimately, regardless of your body "type", the right training and nutrition will make you look more muscular (and mesomorphic). One of the reasons we think there is still some core importance in original body type is that even the most highly developed bodybuilders show hints of their original body. For example, originally endomorphic people tend to look heavier when fully developed and cut, while an ectomorph's smaller joints tend to give away their ectomorphic roots. In bodybuilding terms, when highly developed, endo and meso body types take on a more Herculean (thicker/powerful) aesthetic, whereas ectomorphs lean towards the athletic symmetry of the Apollonian. Note, this is also not considering the impact of any steroid or growth hormone use, which, arguably, could skew the results. We are only interested in natural training here! No matter your type, your training can be adapted to help create the fitness or look you want – although the core features may still be identifiable.

In any case, after you've read the following body type descriptions and have an idea of your closest major body type, it's worth searching online to see some examples of bodies you like that suit your height, size and type to use as an example of what you want to aim for.

ECTOMORPH

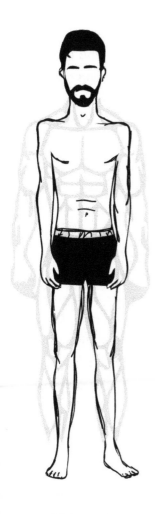

ECTOMORPH
NATURALLY SLIM BUILD
SMALL SKELETAL FRAME

ECTOMORPHS ARE NATURALLY SLIM AND DON'T TEND TO PUT ON WEIGHT EASILY. WHILE BEING SKINNIER THAN AVERAGE CAN BE A DRIVER TO GO TO THE GYM, ECTOMORPHS OFTEN GET THE LEAST MUSCLE BACK FROM TRAINING EFFORT AS THEY ARE FIGHTING AGAINST NATURALLY SLIM GENETICS.

BELOW ARE SOME OF THE CHARACTERISTICS OF A CLASSIC ECTOMORPH:

_LONG LIMBS
_SHORT UPPER BODY
_LONG, NARROW HANDS AND FEET
_NARROWNESS IN CHEST AND
 SHOULDERS
_LITTLE BODY FAT, OR LOW BODY
FAT PERCENTAGE, NATURALLY
_FAST METABOLISM
_MORE DIFFICULTY GAINING
MUSCLE MASS
_SLOWER PHYSICAL
 DEVELOPMENT

Ectomorphs are often referred to as "hard gainers" in bodybuilding circles. Most ectomorphs have difficulty gaining muscle mass and often have to consume more calories, particularly carbohydrates, than other body types to see similar results. Of course, this can be an advantage if you like your pasta, and having a naturally high metabolism means you can get away with a bit more than other body types, particularly endomorphs, who are at the opposite end of the body type scale and find it more difficult to lose fat. Due to the challenge of gaining muscle mass, ectomorphs (particularly in the first few years of training) usually need to do heavy compound exercises, with longer rest periods between sets, to help construct a dense muscle structure. Due to their lower propensity to gain muscle, ectomorphs can sometimes need more recovery time to see progressive gains and are more susceptible to overtraining. Complementing training with cardio work is important and generally healthy, but ectomorphs may have to be careful that they don't do *too much* cardio, as this can slow progress.

It's worth noting again that, unless you are purely ectomorph, you will have other body type characteristics that will show as you train (not to mention as you age) and, as mentioned above, even the most highly trained bodybuilders show signs of their original body type. Interestingly, although Arnold Schwarzenegger – possibly the most famous bodybuilder in the world –

was essentially a mesomorph, he benefited from certain ectomorph characteristics, such as thin joints and waist, which gave him a great Apollonian aesthetic.

It's also worth noting that the reasoning behind the Bigger Brother name came from this concept. The founders of Bigger Brother, despite being both brothers and naturally ectomorphs, of similar height and build, saw differences in their ability to gain muscle mass. Essentially "little brother" is marginally bigger. Regardless of big brother's head start and similar levels of training and diet, little brother soon became *Bigger* Brother!

Here are some examples of famous males with ectomorphic traits:

FRANK ZANE, WILL SMITH, CHANNING TATUM, BRAD PITT, BRUCE LEE, DANIEL CRAIG, FLEX WHEELER, HUGH JACKMAN, CHRIS EVANS, RYAN REYNOLDS, JOE MANGANIELLO, SPIDER-MAN!

Here are some examples of famous females with ectomorphic traits:

THANDIE NEWTON, GISELE BÜNDCHEN, CHERYL (GEORDIE POP STAR), NICOLE SCHERZINGER, JENNIFER ANISTON, EMILY RATAJKOWSKI

MESOMORPH

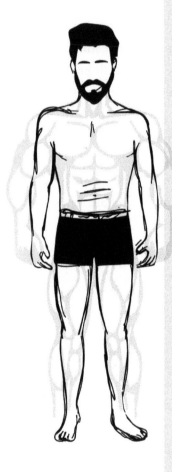

MESOMORPHS ARE WHAT ECTOMORPHS AND ENDOMORPHS CALL "LUCKY BA$*ARDS"! MESOMORPHS USUALLY GET THE MOST EQUAL RESULTS TO THE WORK THEY PUT IN, AS THEIR BODIES ARE MORE NATURALLY GEARED TOWARDS GAINING MUSCLE AND LOSING FAT. HERE ARE SOME OF THE CHARACTERISTICS OF A MESOMORPH:

_LARGE CHEST
_LONG TORSO
_SOLID MUSCLE STRUCTURE
_GREAT STRENGTH
_RECEIVE GREATEST INITIAL BENEFIT FROM TRAINING

MESOMORPH
NATURALLY ATHLETIC BUILD
MEDIUM SKELETAL FRAME

An exact mesomorph usually looks very blocky; solid, with a large head, broad, muscular chest, muscular shoulders and arms, and minimal body fat. As mesomorphs are great candidates for lifting weights, they will benefit from working in a higher rep range than ectomorphs, although a lower range than endomorphs. They can also start including more isolation training in their workouts from quite early on. Although, when we say "isolation", we don't mean training your wrists! Focus on compound movements and certain more isolated movements until fully developed. Meso training will still need to be heavy and hard, but mesomorphs are likely to find gains and progress relatively rapid, with their bodies becoming stronger and bigger in more direct correlation to effort. They are also less susceptible to overtraining than ectomorphs and may find they benefit from more frequent training sessions, although appropriate rest is still important, as for any type.

Due to a mesomorph's natural propensity to gain muscle, it's important to take care in training the body equally (or with focus on the goal "look") as training some body parts more than others could result in uneven development. This is often seen in the gym, where guys have great arms, but lack the shoulders to match, a great chest and skinny legs, or when things look good from the front, but not the back.

It's worth noting that effort and diet is still very important for mesomorphs. They may have the ability to gain lean muscle effectively, but the wrong approach with training, nutrition or rest can also have negative effects. Even a highly developed mesomorph, like Mr. Olympia, Phil Heath, (also known as "The Gift" – due to his genetic gifts for weight training), has to train, eat and rest in the right way for his body type.

Here are some examples of famous males with mesomorphic traits:

ARNOLD SCHWARZENEGGER (ALTHOUGH SOME CLEAR ECTO TRAITS TOO), MICHAEL JOHNSON, PHIL HEATH, ANDRE AGASSI, MIKE TYSON, MAURICE GREENE, MARK WAHLBERG, LOU FERRIGNO, 50 CENT

Here are some examples of famous females with mesomorphic traits:

ALLISON STOKKE, JESSICA BIEL, HALLE BERRY, CINDY CRAWFORD, ANGELA BASSETT, JAMIE EASON, ALICIA MARIE, MADONNA, JENNIFER LAWRENCE (POSSIBLY SOME ENDO TRAITS TOO)

ENDOMORPH

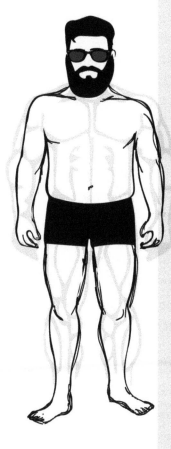

ENDOMORPH
NATURALLY HEAVY BUILD
LARGE SKELETAL FRAME

ENDOMORPHS TIP ECTOMORPHS ON THE OPPOSITE END OF THE SCALE (TERRIBLE PUN, I KNOW!). PEOPLE WHO ARE MORE ENDOMORPHIC ARE NATURALLY HEAVIER AND FIND IT MORE DIFFICULT TO KEEP FAT LEVELS DOWN.

HERE ARE SOME OF THE CHARACTERISTICS OF AN ENDOMORPH:

_**SOFT MUSCULATURE**
_**ROUND FACE**
_**SHORT NECK**
_**WIDE HIPS**
_**SHORTER ARMS AND LEGS**
_**MORE FAT STORAGE**
_**SLOW METABOLISM**
_**DIFFICULTY LOSING FAT**

When it comes to lean muscle mass, endomorphs have almost the exact opposite challenge to ectomorphs, yet some of the muscle-building advantages of mesomorphs. People with endomorphic tendencies are likely to find that their strength and overall size increases relatively easily with weight lifting. However, of the three categories, they will most likely need to do more endurance work in a higher rep range, with lower rest times, more cardio and careful dieting, to keep their propensity to gain fat weight under control.

People with more endomorphic traits may find they need to include longer/more cardio sessions within their training plans, and eat even more carefully, in comparison to the other categories. A diet with controlled calories, yet essential nutrition for desired size, will be of particular importance. On the plus side, endomorphs have the advantage of having a very dense (heavy looking) muscle structure, even when cut. For this reason, it's not that surprising that many of the biggest and most powerful looking Mr. Olympias have had endomorphic traits. Like ectomorphs, they may also find a compelling drive to go to the gym, although for opposite reasons.

Here are some examples of famous males with endomorphic traits:

DWAYNE "THE ROCK" JOHNSON, RUSSELL CROWE, DR DRE, DAVE DRAPER, JACK BLACK, VING RHAMES, DORIAN YATES (ALTHOUGH STRONG MESO CHARACTERISTICS AS WELL), LEE PRIEST

Here are some examples of famous females with endo-morphic traits:

JENNIFER LOPEZ, BEYONCÉ, KIM KARDASHIAN, KATE WINSLET, SOFÍA VERGARA, SOPHIE DAHL, NIGELLA LAWSON, MEGHAN TRAINOR, OPRAH WINFREY

BODY TYPE TARGETS

As highlighted, somatotypes – or body typing generally – should not be taken too literally. We are all different and although we tend to have certain characteristics, each one of us has advantages and disadvantages. The key is to understand your body as well as possible – so you can adapt your training to maximise your advantages and reduce the barriers of your disadvantages.

For example, mesomorphs may have a tendency to gain lean muscle, but they can often be quite blocky and square in appearance. Depending on desired look, mesomorphs may have to adapt their training to bring out certain body areas. Ectomorphs will have difficulty gaining muscle, but once they gain some base mass, it is easier to stay lean and can look more aesthetically pleasing in terms of general opinion. Endomorphs may be challenged by fat loss but will find it easier to look particularly massive (even when lean) next to a meso-morph or ectomorph. As mentioned above, a number of the biggest bodybuilders and wrestlers (e.g. Dwayne

Johnson) could be considered to have endomorphic tendencies.

Looking at the success of some of the world's most famous bodies, Bigger Brother thinks there is no all-encompassing body type limitation on achieving a great body with the right effort and nutrition; although it's good to focus on achieving a target that is matched to your body. In other words (and discounting drugs), if you're very skinny and under six feet tall, it's unlikely that you will be able to look like The Rock, or Lou Ferrigno in his prime, but perhaps you could develop your body to look like Zac Efron, Tyrese Gibson or Frank Zane (if you don't know who he is, have a look on Google).

Similarly, if you're over six feet two and endomorphic, you might find it harder to look like Hugh Jackman's Wolverine, but you might have a shot at looking like The Rock! The most important thing is to set targets that work for you and adapt training and nutrition to meet your goals.

RESISTANCE TRAINING FOR BEGINNERS
(& Everyone Else)

FITNESS, GYM & OTHER MYTHS

- ☑ **THE QUALITY OF THE GYM IS EQUAL TO THE PRICE AND NUMBER OF FANCY MACHINES AVAILABLE.** You do not need a fancy gym to develop fitness and a great physique.

- ☑ **LIFTING WEIGHTS WILL TURN YOU INTO A MUSCLE-BOUND MONSTER.** Even for the most genetically gifted, weight training for strength and size takes time, it doesn't happen overnight (not even with help from science).

- ☑ **WEIGHT TRAINING AND BODYBUILDING IS FOR JOCKS, NOT SKINNY OR CHUBBY GEEKS.** Not looking naturally lean and/or muscular is often a key driver for people to start going to the gym.

- ☑ **THE BIG GUYS IN THE GYM KNOW THE MOST ABOUT WEIGHT TRAINING.** While some might, it's a dangerous assumption, as genetics can play a major part in lean mass. The guys who have to work harder for results are often the ones who have built up a wide knowledge base.

☑ **HAVING MUSCLE MAKES YOU FIT.** It does, to a degree, but cardio is important to overall fitness.

☑ **GENETICS DON'T MATTER, ALL YOU HAVE TO DO IS WORK HARD.** Hard work is key, but genetics go a long way. Athletes' success stories, like those of Michael Phelps, Arnold Schwarzenegger and Usain Bolt, involved hard work, and that, combined with some natural genetics, allowed them to go further than many with a similar work ethic.

☑ **GOING TO THE GYM EVERYDAY WILL MAKE YOUR MUSCLES GROW.** Not necessarily. Over-training muscles can be detrimental to your training.

☑ **CURLING FOR BIG BICEPS, EQUALS BIG ARMS.** Biceps are relatively small muscles in comparison to other body parts, including triceps. Compound movements are key and hitting the three heads of the triceps can be far more effective at increasing arm size.

☑ **FAT IS CONVERTED TO MUSCLE AND MUSCLE BECOMES FAT.** Fat or muscle is lost or gained. The illusion of the conversion is in loss of muscle and gaining of fat, due to lack of muscle stimulation and poor diet (and vice versa).

☑ **WEIGHT TRAINING IN YOUR TEENS STUNTS GROWTH**. The research suggests that this is highly unlikely and there are lots of examples of people who have trained in their teens and seen no detrimental effects to height. This myth may be more prominent because it would seem that a lot of champion bodybuilders are less than six feet tall!

☑ **LUNCH IS FOR WIMPS AND SLEEPING IS FOR LOSERS**. Oh, if only I had £1 for every time someone has said one of these phrases in a macho display in the office! No, no, no – sing it like Dawn Penn! – this couldn't be more wrong. Eating (appropriately) and sleep are for athletes, sportsmen and anyone who wants a fit, healthy and strong body and mind.

☑ **IN ORDER TO LOSE WEIGHT, GET LEAN AND FIT, I MUST EAT LESS**. This is not necessarily true, as exercising and eating too little of the right calories for your level of physical activity can negatively impact progress.

BIGGER BROTHER GYM DOS & DON'TS

☑   Don't let your phone distract you. Better yet, leave your phone behind – you're in the gym to train, not check your Facebook, Twitter and Snapchat, or WhatsApp your girlfriend/boyfriend. If you really want to use the latest gym app, fine, but keep the smartphone distractions to a minimum. Best solution, get some wearable tech to track progress and leave your phone in the locker.

☑   Keep it simple – it's not necessary to have fancy clothing, equipment and tech.

     ▪ If you must take your own music and phone/player then make sure it's well out of the way and don't fiddle with it during your training. Have it ready, so it lasts your training session without any need for adjustment.

     ▪ Don't bother with fancy gym clothes. Trainers, shorts and T-shirts are all you need, it's not a fashion show.

     ▪ Straps, supports and other extras. Unless you've built the foundations and are on course to be the next body pro or have been advised by a doctor, you don't need extra stuff.

- If, like me, the metal and sweat can give you a rash and you'd prefer not to be slimed, there's no harm in wearing gloves, but ensure they are thin, light gloves that don't support or pad the hands too much. You want your hands, fingers and palms to get stronger, as they are your levers for the weights – so let them get a workout. You might even find that when you are training in a new way or to a new level, your hands give out before the muscle you are training and your hands are sore for a few days after. This is OK, because it means they'll get stronger and support you in working your other muscles harder the next time.

- Take a towel; no one wants your slime on the gym bench and you don't want to lie in their slime either.

☑ If you see guys doing crossover flys and other fancier moves, don't assume you need to do that too, to get in shape or have a great body. Gyms nowadays are equipped with all kinds of fancy apparatus. The 1960s and early 1970s was perhaps the Golden Age of Bodybuilding. It was the time of Reg Park, Arnie, Lou Ferrigno, Serge Nubret, Franco Columbu, Sergio Oliva, Frank Zane and more. It was the end of an era, when the Apollonian aesthetics were still as important as anatomy and size in the top bodybuilding world. Many would have got to their 200–245lb (90–110kg) lean, sculpted mass without any fancy equipment or fancy gyms. Part of the reason Arnie became so impressive, so young, is he was influenced by powerlifting moves. Franco Columbu was a powerlifter, which helped him become a legendary bodybuilder in the shorter man category. He could also blow up a hot water bottle, but that's by the by. The key thing is, power-lifting moves and other compound core moves can help develop a very powerful, lean, balanced physique, without fancy apparatus. One of my most successful periods of muscle/strength growth was when I didn't have a gym, just a few dumbbells in the garage. I started inventing variants of what I would have done in the gym, and did things like upside down push-ups with my feet against the wall.

☑ Don't spend too much time (or don't even bother) doing isolation moves until you have gained sufficient mass using core moves – particularly wrist curls! :)

☑ Don't train body parts unevenly. Be what Bigger Brother calls a "Symmitarian"!

☑ Don't drink calorie dense supplements. If you've had the right supplements before and after, this should be sufficient. I also can't understand how it would be possible to exercise properly and with appropriate intensity while digesting!

☑   Don't drink fancy energy drinks while you train. Plain water is fine and you should ensure you are well-hydrated throughout. Having a bottle of water is good, but not essential. Technically, there isn't really a need to carry a bottle when the gym has water fountains. After a section of training, or a move to another section of the gym, a quick trip to the water fountain means you're not sitting around between sets. If you have any issues with hydration and cramping you could also try adding electrolytes in your water to see if that helps.

☑   Stay focused. Ignore the other people in the gym and what they are doing, concentrate on what you need to do. Be a machine, be a robot. Push distractions out of your mind and think only about the moves, your stretching, breathing, lifting, tensing, muscle contractions and pump. Not only will this improve your training, but it will also help you switch off from the stresses of life.

☑   Don't be afraid to stretch muscles as you train. It's amazing how few people do this. Think it's girlie to stretch? Think again.

☑   Be prepared and have a clear idea of the training you are going to do before you go to the gym.

GROUNDWORK TRAINING

NOTE: THIS SECTION IS FOR PEOPLE WHO ARE STARTING OUT OR GETTING BACK INTO EXERCISE AFTER LONG PERIODS (SIX MONTHS+) WITHOUT ANY FORM OF RESISTANCE TRAINING. IT CAN ALSO BE TREATED AS AN OPPORTUNITY TO RESET YOUR TRAINING, TAKE A BREAK FROM THE GYM AND/OR REIGNITE YOUR MOTIVATION.

Before you go rushing into the gym (or back to the gym) and picking up the heaviest weight you can lift or, alternatively, picking up some light weights and just going through the motions, remember the words of Mr Miyagi, Daniel-san's sensei in the 1980's movie, *The Karate Kid*: "Wax on, wax off!" If you don't know the movie, you can view the clip here: BIT.LY/WAXONOFF

Why is this relevant? Well, because it highlights the importance of doing the basics first and establishing a foundation.

In the movie, Daniel (Ralph Macchio) wants Mr Miyagi (Noriyuki "Pat" Morita) to teach him karate, so Miyagi gets Daniel to perform boring chores around his house, like waxing cars, sanding the floor, painting the fence/house, etc. Each activity has a specific movement which must be performed accurately – like circular hand motions and precise up and down arm, wrist to hand movements.

Daniel fails to see any connection between the chores and his training. After doing them for some time, he confronts Mr Miyagi in frustration, thinking he's just being tricked into doing work for him. In response, Mr Miyagi throws out some offensive karate moves and, to Daniel's surprise, he blocks them using exactly the techniques he was using to wax, sand and paint. Without even realising it, Daniel had developed muscle memory and learned core defensive movements. These basic movements were the groundwork for his karate training.

So, the moral of the story is, take some time to do some groundwork. Not only will it prepare you for advancing your training, it can also give you some base strength (even size) or allow you to regain some base strength that will make starting or getting back into training much more manageable. Also, you don't have to do your groundwork in the gym. You could do it at home, in your garden, in a park or anywhere you like. So, if you haven't got your gym subscription yet, why not save yourself a month's fees and spend the money on some good high-quality food to help with your training instead? If you've already got the membership, but haven't been using it enough, get back in there to make up for those wasted payments!

As a beginner, or to reset your training, it's advisable to do the conditioning training for a minimum of six weeks, or at least until you can do a reasonable number of reps, in total, per move, in the conditioning workout.

Why? The simple answer is, there is no point in using a weight if you can't lift your own body weight a reasonable number of times.

If, after six weeks, you still feel you need a bit more time, there is no harm in continuing the conditioning phase for a longer period. The key thing is, the more you have mastered the conditioning phase, the more confident you will be and the easier it will be to maximise the advantages, including early gains of a weight training beginner (or restarter).

The first time I went in the gym, when I was in my late teens, it was a disaster. I wasted lots of time doing all the wrong things and saw little benefit. In fact, I seemed to lose strength and ability. This, I now know, was down to poor understanding of nutrition, recovery and lack of training knowledge.

Two years later, when I tried again and went to the gym with friends, I started to read extensively about training. Then, training with weights, or "bodybuilding", or even going to a gym with real iron was less mainstream than it is now, but if you looked around you could find useful sources of information. This time I was more prepared and I already had a reasonable level of exercise experience and body weight conditioning from rollerblading, running, swimming, and even surfing (well, mainly paddling). So, once a few basics were understood, the gym became a regular thing, and after a few months and some hard work, I saw gains that made friends notice and ask how I did it. Some friends even assumed I had the "right genetics" but, unfortunately, as a hard-gaining skinny dude, it wasn't the case!

NOTABLY, MY FRIEND GROUP WHILE AT UNIVERSITY OFTEN WENT TO THE GYM AT SIMILAR TIMES TO ME, BUT NEVER SAW THE SAME RESULTS. DUE TO MY MUSCLE PROGRESS ADVANCING ME FROM A SKINNY 67KG TO A LEAN, MUSCULAR 87KG OVER ABOUT TWO AND A BIT YEARS, PLUS MY COMMITMENT TO REGULAR TRAINING, I GOT THE NICKNAME "GYM BOY". THE REALITY OF THIS IS THERE WAS NO SECRET SAUCE, I JUST READ MORE, TRAINED MORE INTENSELY, ATE BETTER THAN THEY DID AND ADAPTED WHERE I SAW RESULTS.

When I returned to resistance training after my big mistake (or "just being lazy" period) in my early 30s, I wasn't going to make these mistakes again. This time, I started with the groundwork essentially as it's outlined in this book.

Once you are confident you've mastered conditioning or have got yourself back into base condition, you're ready for weights.

BUILDING: MASS TRAINING

"Wait!" you shout. "Isn't this book called *The 'Lean' Exec*? I'm not looking to gain lots of muscle and look like a bodybuilder. Why are you telling me about mass training? I don't want to spend endless hours in the gym, training to be one of those massive overblown dudes. I just want to be lean, healthy and athletic."

Well, doing a bit of mass training isn't going to turn you into the Hulk. Certainly not in the short term and without the appropriate diet, but gaining is very useful if you want some fat-fighting muscle and to reap the benefits of strength when it comes to weight loss. If it works for Jeff Bezos, the founder and CEO of Amazon, it can work for you. ;)

One of the most important books I ever read was Arnold Schwarzenegger's *Encyclopaedia of Modern Bodybuilding*. It's about three inches thick, has a gazillion pages, weighs a ton (for a book) and talks about huge guys lifting incredible weights, and even how to perfect your posing in skimpy trunks. Now, it's never been my ambition to be a bodybuilder of that proportion, or to pose in skimpy trunks, for that matter, but the principles can certainly help guide success, whatever your goal.

Learning what makes you stronger and grows muscle is important, as having trained muscles makes your training far more effective and efficient when you do it. And, again, a reminder: it's not about losing or gaining "weight" as such, and it's not about "converting" muscle to fat. It's about *building* muscle and *burning* fat – this is what changes your body composition and helps you balance life as a Lean Exec.

Almost every time I go to the gym I see guys, girls and even PTs wasting their time and wondering why they never see results (part of the reason to write this book!). Skinny guys doing endless reps and supersets, wondering why they aren't gaining strength and/or muscle. Heavyset guys wondering why, despite their strength, they don't have the girls drooling over them, like they do over the athletic guy over there, who isn't as strong.

One of the big issues is that most of the training plans and information available is either middle of the road or "fitness model", "bodybuilder", "celebrity" or quick "weight loss" training. This can work, and it's not to say that some of it's not good or useful, but it can be confusing and isn't always suitable for normal life. As an example, if you Google "Arnold Schwarzenegger workout" you get his famous split routine, which was two and a half hours in the morning and two and a half hours in the afternoon, six days per week! Without already being a bodybuilder, having some gifted genetics, having the time in a day or even taking steroids, this is unrealistic for most mere mortals.

It's almost impossible to find details of Arnold's early training, although he touches on it in his autobiography.

The truth is, Arnold had an incredible physique (even by today's standards) before he ever trained using this routine, which includes a range of isolation movements. His foundations were built in powerlifting-style training in Graz, which most likely included very little other than squats, deadlifts and bench presses, then perhaps cleans, rows and barbell curls. Again, though, the reference is not so you can turn yourself into a 100kg bodybuilder (unless you want to), but that the application of some of the core techniques will help you develop your body in the desired way and as you see fit (pardon the pun).

These moves, often referred to as "Power Training", are also important to build up dense, hard muscle mass, the kind of fat burning muscle that looks solid, thick and powerful. Including these power moves in your training also helps to break plateaus and bring on hypertrophy, where the muscles become bigger and stronger. These core, compound, multi-joint movements are technically all you need to do in a gym to construct a man mountain. So, put down the cables and the fancy ball, drop the wrist curls and the complicated supersets, and let's go back to basics and PUMP some IRON!

NOTE: A LOT OF PEOPLE DON'T UNDERSTAND GYMS. HOW CAN YOU GET ENJOYMENT OUT OF MONOTONOUSLY LIFTING SOME WEIGHTS? BIGGER BROTHER BELIEVES THIS HAS A LOT TO DO WITH MIND-SET, COMBINED WITH INTENSITY, AND NOT APPRECIATING THE BENEFITS QUICKLY ENOUGH DUE TO LACK OF KNOWLEDGE AND

EXPERIENCE. THOSE PEOPLE THAT GET PAST THIS INITIAL THINK-ING AND SEE THE ESCAPISM, PURPOSE AND ALMOST MEDITATIVE BENEFITS OF WEIGHT TRAINING UNDERSTAND THIS, NOT TO MEN-TION THE ADDICTIVE, POSITIVE FEELING OF "THE PUMP". THESE CORE COMPOUND MOVEMENTS SPEED UP THE PROCESS, WITH THE RIGHT EATING AND SLEEP ALLOWING YOU TO TRULY FEEL AND SEE THE BENEFITS MUCH FASTER. ALSO, DUE TO THEIR MULTI-JOINT ENGAGEMENT, THEY ARE EXCELLENT AT BURNING UP THE FAT!

SIZE, STRENGTH & STRENGTH ENDURANCE

There are lots of theories and research into what is the best way to build muscle size and strength. While the results and beliefs on techniques can vary, one aspect is pretty much universal. In order to gain strength, size and/or endurance, muscles must be pushed beyond their current capacity. Essentially, the muscle fibre is broken down with training and reformed, stronger, which in principle translates into bigger and/or better (hypertrophy – see definition below) in rest periods.

HYPERTROPHY

/HAHY-PUR-TRUH-FEE/

NOUN, PLURAL HYPERTROPHIES.

Enlargement of a part, organ or tissue; excessive growth.

This is why it's very important to understand that training itself does not increase the size, strength or endurance of muscles, necessarily; it's the combination of recuperation and nutrition that accompanies the training that allows the muscle to increase. Here's another useful quote I found with a search online:

ONE HOUR THREE TIMES PER WEEK IN THE GYM IS NO COUNTERBALANCE TO ALL OF THE OTHER BEHAVIOUR IN THOSE OTHER 165 HOURS.

MARK TWIGHT, GYM JONES

Essentially, unless you are very genetically gifted or using steroids, if you train the same muscles every day, but don't fuel up or sleep to match the level of training, they would be unlikely to grow or improve as they would not have the time to recover and get stronger/ better. In fact, you might even find the opposite, with the muscles getting weaker, because they have not recovered enough or are malnourished. However, the more advanced you become, the better your muscles are likely to become at recovering. Highly trained muscles recover from fatigue faster than untrained muscles.

NOTE: IT'S OFTEN ASSUMED THAT ANABOLIC STEROIDS MAKE MUSCLES GROW AND INCREASE. WHAT STEROIDS (A SYNTHETIC VERSION OF THE HORMONE TESTOSTERONE) ACTUALLY DO IS ALLOW THE PERSON TAKING THE STEROIDS TO RECOVER/

IMPROVE MORE QUICKLY FROM THEIR TRAINING. THEY HELP THE BODY'S MUSCLE PRODUCE MORE PROTEIN, SO THAT WITH TRAINING, MUSCLES CAN INCREASE IN SIZE, STRENGTH AND ATHLETIC PERFORMANCE MORE EASILY. ANABOLIC STEROIDS ALSO ALLOW THE BODY TO PRODUCE MORE ADENOSINE TRI-PHOSPHATE (ATP), THE FUEL MUSCLES NEED TO CONTRACT/MOVE. RESEARCH SUGGESTS IT ALLOWS MORE FREQUENT BREAKDOWN AND RECOVERY IN THE SHORT TERM BUT CAN HAVE LONG-TERM NEGATIVE EFFECTS TO THE NATURAL ABILITY FOR MUSCLE TO HEAL. BIGGER BROTHER DOESN'T USE OR CONDONE USING STEROIDS!

In consideration of what brings on hypertrophy, thought also needs to be given to "types" of strength and fitness. A sprinter might be very fit and able to run 100 metres in under 10 seconds, but they might struggle to compete with a light, lean marathon runner in a long race of endurance. Similarly, one athlete may be able to lift 500lbs once, while another athlete may not be able to lift 500lbs, but be able to lift their body weight over and over again for longer periods of time. This is the difference between strength and strength endurance. Ultimately, resistance training and fitness requires a combination of both types of strength, although how much of each type will play a role in how the body looks.

Looking at the most advanced level of strength sport, a strong man like Hafþór Júlíus Björnsson (The Mountain in *Game of Thrones*) who can lift over 425kg

(936lbs) twice!! is super-strong. His main aim is to lift the heaviest weight possible – for only one or a few reps. Therefore, endurance is less important, it's all about raw power and there isn't really an advantage for him to be too lean, which shows when looking at his massive body (with some endomorphic traits). At the opposite end of the scale you have gymnasts or calisthenics athletes, who look muscular, but are very light and lean (ectomorphic and mesomorphic traits), as they need to use strength endurance to hold their bodies for longer periods or lift their bodies multiple times.

Bodybuilders have to mix both of these types of strength to combine the size and lean muscle development of an advanced, highly trained individual. They use very heavy weight and lift it for relatively high reps, combining raw strength with strength endurance – although only with the right mix (for their own unique body), so that it's not detrimental to the aesthetic they are looking to achieve. The key thing with bodybuilders is that they have worked their way up to such significant strength that their workouts would seem like strength exercise to mere mortals, but as they are doing higher rep ranges it is actually also applying strength endurance.

Why is all of this important? It's important because many bog-standard training programmes prescribe standardised reps per set and often include lots of isolation movements and cardio. This is great if your genetics mean anything you do makes your muscles advance (although it's still not necessarily right) or you are already about the size and strength you want to be and need to focus on leaning up and sculpting certain aspects of your body. For everyone else, this can help improve your body, but it won't necessarily help you get to your specific goals as fast. In fact, in some cases it can restrict your growth, because your body is quite clever at adapting (even for those whose bodies change more slowly) and conserving energy for what it thinks you need to do.

Let's go back to our runner example. If you go for lots of long distance (10k+) runs (aerobic exercise) numerous times per week, you can eat significant calories and yet there is a high chance your body will still shrink down to be slender and lighter. This is because your body is not only using the calories, but also being sent messages that it needs to be able to carry you for long distances and having extra weight is not helpful for this. Therefore, the body breaks down molecules (catabolism) and even cannibalises muscle to release energy to meet the needs of the endurance exercise. On the other hand, if you regularly do short sprints (anaerobic exercise), using all your power for very short bursts, with a rest between each burst, your body realises it needs more power and muscle to shift the body across the short distance. This is because this anaerobic exercise triggers restriction of oxygen to muscles, which is beneficial for non-endurance athletes like sprinters and bodybuilders, to increase anabolism, muscle mass and fat loss.

There is lots of research out there, and a quick search online will verify this and provide greater detail, but unless you want to know the science, all you have to do to understand or see this concept is to look at the difference between the body of a professional marathon runner and that of a sprinter. If you want to be more muscular, like a sprinter, then too much endurance (long distance cardio) marathon running or cycling type exercise is going to restrict your ability to develop that form. Furthermore, if your goal is to gain strength/mass, it makes more sense to focus on lower repetition heavy training, with longer rest periods, than lots of reps with short rest periods. Reps can increase once you have gained the initial strength.

As mentioned above, there are many theories about which techniques work and which ones don't work to encourage hypertrophy, increase ability and/or make improvements in training. Bigger Brother believes through reading, research and experience over 20 years that outside of genetics, nutrition and rest, the following points are good laws to stick by:

☑   Extreme endurance training (e.g. long distance running and cycling) = very slim, ectomorphic body characteristics.

- ☑ Pure strength training (e.g. World's Strongest Man, Olympic lifts) = extreme strength, usually large, with some endomorphic body characteristics.

- ☑ Strength endurance (e.g. sprinters, Hollywood actors trained for superhero roles) = above-average strength, with mesomorphic body characteristics – size and look dependent on training emphasis.

- ☑ High strength plus strength endurance (e.g. bodybuilder) = high strength, with extreme mesomorphic body characteristics.

- ☑ To have strength endurance, strength plus strength endurance, or a body in this range sooner, it helps to focus on increasing strength first.

These are, of course, rules of thumb; they are not completely exact as there are too many variables, but the key is to focus on balancing the training towards the activity that will deliver the results you want. For example, one or two 5–10k runs a week may not impact your growth, if the other 80%–90% of the time you are training and eating for muscle growth. However, if you spend eight hours a week in the gym, lifting a weight for 25 reps a set, and run the best part of two marathons a week, you're unlikely to increase your lean mass. Most likely, you will cannibalise any fat-fighting muscle.

Alternatively, lifting heavy weights for no more than 5–8 reps, combined with interval training for 20–30 mins a few days a week is likely to get you strong and lean. Bigger Brother has found that some of the best training for increasing strength and size rapidly, as well as breaking plateaus, is to do core compound movements, like deadlifts and squats, once per week, for 10 sets, with a weight that you can only lift 1–3 times a set and ensuring you have two minutes rest between each set. When you do this correctly, to your max, it feels like your whole body has delayed onset of muscle soreness (DOMS) for days and, as long as you eat and rest well, your body has little it can do, but grow stronger to compensate. While this may be too extreme for regular activity in normal daily life, hopefully it illustrates the idea.

TIPS FOR STRENGTH TRAINING

☑ Try doing 4 heavy sets of low reps (1–3) including a drop set of 6–8 reps, following the 3rd and 4th sets of an exercise. Ensure you rest for a longer period, like 90 seconds to 2 minutes (avoid more than 2 minutes) between sets, to ensure you can recoup energy to lift the next set.

☑ Go back to basics: try doing a power move session once per week, focused on low rep (1–3), high set training. For example, do 6-10 sets of deadlifts (or 4-5 sets of deadlifts and 3-5 sets of squats) using a weight you can only lift with good form 1-3 times per set. Rest for around 90 seconds to 2 minutes between sets. This should be all you need to do in the session and should take around 40-45 minutes to complete.

WARNINGS: IT'S IMPORTANT THAT YOU USE GOOD FORM AT ALL TIMES. THESE MOVES CAN CAUSE SEVERE INJURY IF DONE IN-CORRECTLY. START LIGHT AND TEST YOUR STRENGTH OVER A FEW SESSIONS BEFORE ATTEMPTING ANYTHING TOO DRAMAT-IC. IN ADDITION, THIS TRAINING CAN HIT YOUR NERVOUS SYS-TEM VERY HARD, AND IT CAN GIVE YOU DOMS FOR DAYS AFTER-WARDS, SO YOU MIGHT WANT TO FOLLOW THIS WITH A PURE REST DAY. BE MINDFUL THAT YOU EAT AND SLEEP WELL, TO RECOVER EFFECTIVELY, AND IT CAN BE A USEFUL TECHNIQUE FOR INCREASING STRENGTH, SIZE AND BREAK PLATEAUS.

☑   Once you've completed your usual reps on a set and can't lift another rep, put down the weight for 10-15 seconds, then pick it up again and try to do 1-3 more reps. Even if you can't lift a whole rep, lift it as far as you can and hold it, so the muscle is tense, and lower it back slowly. You can also try doing a drop set straight after, although don't drop the weight too much; enough to do a couple of reps should be enough.

☑ Try different rep ranges. For example, if you've been training with under 5 reps, try training for a few weeks with a lower weight and 6–10 rep range. You can also try higher rep ranges, although generally, once you get over 10 reps a set, you're focusing more and more on strength endurance (see the section on strength versus strength endurance earlier in the book).

☑ Cheating. Generally, Bigger Brother recommends avoiding cheating on an exercise, but there are times when it can be strategically useful to help push your muscles beyond their current limits. By "cheating", we mean using your body motion and other muscles to "throw the weight" up with control, so you can deliver a few extra partial, forced and/or negative reps with a weight you can't lift anymore with full range of motion/good form. You could also ask a gym partner to help you push the weight up a few more times, although Bigger Brother is not a huge fan of this as your partner may not know exactly how much help you need and may overcompensate. Cheats can work well for moves like bicep curls, where you have exhausted the biceps on a weight and can't lift any more with full range of motion and good form. In this case, you use your shoulders and body movement to get the weight up as far as you need to complete a rep, or to get to the top of the curl position, so you can lower the weight slowly (negative rep) to put additional tension on the muscles. Another example is when you're doing dips or pull-ups and can't do anymore; you then jump up or use a "step" to help you get into a position from where you can finish another rep or do a negative rep (lower your body down, in this case). Bigger Brother is a big fan of using a bit of cheating to do some forced and negative reps at the end of sets of body weight exercises. Generally, we only recommend using cheating techniques at the end of sets and sessions where you are trying to push your muscles and have already completed your core reps and sets with good form.

☑ Try slow, very controlled repetitions, which keep the pressure on for longer. You could mix these with normal speed repetitions. The trick will be intensity, so focus on what makes your muscles work hardest.

☑ On the first set of every exercise (after a warm up) do a weight you can only lift 1 time, with good form. Try to lift it a 2nd time without cheating and hold it for a few seconds at the farthest point you can get to. For sets 2 and 3, use a weight where you can do 6 good reps. On the 4th set, complete

5–6 reps and do a drop set for 2–4 reps (you should fail to complete by or before 4 reps). You could also do this with a 5th set that repeats set 4. Experiment with different rest times between sets, but as a general rule of thumb you might want to give yourself 1 minute 15 seconds to 2 minutes' rest between sets. Try to avoid longer rest times, even when the focus is on strength and muscle growth.

☑ Changing split training (usually for experienced people training more than 3 times per week). If you've been splitting your body parts in each session one way for a couple of months, try changing the split. For example, if you have been doing chest, shoulders and triceps one day and back and biceps another, you could change the split to chest and back one day and shoulders and arms another.

☑ Keep training focused, intense and under 1 hour – ideally 45-60 minutes.

☑ If you're eating enough of the right macronutrients and calories, but still not gaining the way you want, then beyond upping your clean calorie intake, it's worth experimenting with some of the following:

- Cut down cardio (and walking) during the week. Too much cardio could be burning up more calories than you think.

- If you're doing more than 3 days (3 hours) of training per week, try dropping to 3 days a week with 2 days' rest in between sessions. Make sure the 3 hours are intense though.

- Increase intensity by cutting rest, increasing reps, sets and/or weight, before you consider starting to increase session time.

- Try taking a week off from training and let your body settle, with full rest. It does no harm to take a week off as frequently as every 5–8 weeks. As long as you continue to eat well and do some low impact activity, it's unlikely to upset your progress and may even help you gain.

A NOTE ON STRENGTH TRAINING NUTRITION

As important as it is to lift the right weights to gain mass, nutrition is equally important. If you don't eat enough of the right calories to fuel the growth, you can actually see strength loss, not just strength gain. Depending on your size, the size you want to be and how fast you want to get there, for best results you are most likely going to need to eat 2,500 to as much as 5,000 good clean quality calories, with the right balance of macronutrients (macros) daily to reach your goals. More specifics on nutrition in the Diet & Nutrition chapter.

SCULPTING A MASTERPIECE

As you gain, and reach the size and strength level you want, it may become more important to increase isolation movements. For most people, this doesn't mean breaking down your routines into epic multi-isolation exercises and multiple, long drawn out sessions. If you have been generally good at keeping your calorie intake balanced and in control in relation to your training effort and have considered the avoidance of weak points (more on these later in the book), then even mass training should already have sculpted an athletic, symmetrical, muscular build in a below average body fat range.

NOTE: IF YOU ARE SKINNY TO START WITH, IT'S NORMAL TO HOLD OR GAIN A BIT OF FAT WHEN INCREASING MUSCLE STRENGTH AND SIZE – PARTICULARLY AS THE EXTRA CALORIES HELP (NOTE THE POINT EARLIER ABOUT STRONG MEN TRAINING FOR RAW POWER). THE MORE CAREFULLY YOU WATCH THE TYPE OF CALORIES YOU CONSUME, THE LESS FAT YOU WILL GAIN. IF YOU'RE OVERWEIGHT, MASS TRAINING WITH THE RIGHT NUTRITION CAN ALSO TRIM YOU DOWN.

The idea that you need to do lots of fancy moves and exercises to build a lean muscular physique is a fallacy. In the early days of bodybuilding, legends like Steve Reeves (often referenced for his ideal body measurements) built a 210lb (95kg) sculpture (naturally), using around 15 free weight exercises. Similarly, the simple 5x5 training of Reg Park (also a Hollywood Hercules, like Steve Reeves) is enough to build spectacular size and shape. You might not want to be as big as Steve Reeves or Reg Park, but until you have built an impressive fit physique at the size you want, you don't need to get complicated. If you get to this level and want to take it further, great, go for it! By then, you should know your body very well, in which case you should be evolving your training to fit your goals (and be beyond this book).

Although it's possible to shape a fantastic body with only a few moves, there are some considerations, and Bigger Brother isn't totally against varying workouts. The reason we stress the importance of not over-complicating is we believe that there are a lot of messages (particularly sales messages) out there about fitness and sometimes the truth can get lost in the clutter.

With regard to varying workouts, the reality is, we are all different and different muscles can develop differently for each individual – even in the case of the author's, and another reference to the Bigger Brother concept. One brother finds it easier to develop the size and strength of the pull muscles (particularly biceps) while the other finds the chest and triceps (push muscles) develop more easily.

Therefore, even though The Lean Exec training methods are designed to maintain symmetry, it is important to keep in mind the natural tendencies of your body (which you will notice along the way). If you follow the training methods, the differences will be minimised, but you will need to consider avoiding weak points and also compensating for body parts that may need some additional attention.

AVOIDING WEAK POINTS

We all have strengths and weaknesses in our physiology, as well as mentally. The discipline of regular training can be very good for developing both the body and mind to be stronger, although in training you will soon discover (if you haven't already) weak points that you need to develop and most likely work harder on so they match the rest of your progress. For example, two similarly strong and muscular people can look quite different. One may have a wider back and strong shoulders, while the other may have larger arms.

In the case of the author and his Bigger Brother, particular weaknesses included calves and biceps for one and triceps and chest for the other. It affects most of us, to some degree. If you do a quick search online you can find details about how Arnold Schwarzenegger terminated his calf weakness. Now, you may not be competing for Mr. Olympia or aiming to be a fitness model, but you want to look balanced, as having good biceps looks a lot better alongside equally muscular triceps, shoulders, chest, back and legs, whatever the size. It will also help to make your strength more balanced and develop overall practical fitness.

To avoid seeing your weak points slip behind and your body look unbalanced, keep an eye on your development and note the difference in performance across different body parts. This should be quite apparent and it's not vain to monitor this with a mirror, it's just sensible to avoid looking... well, odd. Below are some techniques you can use to help avoid weak points:

☑ Include power moves that will develop the overall body. Moves like deadlifts, squats and military presses are known to help increase overall body fitness, strength and mass.

☑ Focus the core of your workouts on compound movements which engage multiple muscle groups. Ensure your training plan includes compound movements that cover all the body parts across your workouts each week. Be sure to train body parts with equal consistency each week. Regular strong chest workouts coupled with lacklustre back workouts are likely to produce unbalanced results.

☑ Use good form with every exercise and don't cheat, just to look like you can lift more weight. For example, it's important to do bicep curls with a strict movement. It's easy to get lazy and put the elbows too far forward and/or swing the weight, which will engage your deltoids (shoulders) more than your arms. Keep elbows straight and pinned to your sides.

☑ Priority principle: do compound movements first, unless you are seeing a major lag in a muscle/ muscle group. In other words, it's better not to start with isolation movements, but if you are seeing a lag, start with one of the isolation movements, then do the compound movements, then finish with the remaining isolation movements. However, this should be the exception for people who are on the way to intermediate training or who are experienced and have been training long enough to see weak points to correct. Also, isolation movement doesn't mean fancy moves or training your fingers – stick to the core moves!

A WORD ON CUTTING TRAINING

If your goal is super-lean aesthetics, for fastest results with weight training, it's usually best to focus on strength and mass (bulking) first, and then cutting. Trying to do both at the same time can make for a slow process and can be detrimental to progress. This is why you often hear in the media about actors eating 5,000 calories and lifting heavy weights, then dieting strictly, when in training for a major role where they need to look built, but lean, in six months. Think Hugh Jackman for

Wolverine, Henry Cavill for Superman, Mark Wahlberg for Pain & Gain, Ben Affleck for Batman or "The Rock" for everything! Slow, steady development (or maintenance mode) is only really useful for someone who is already within a few kilos of their ideal/desired size.

NOTE: TO MAKE THE CUTTING PROCESS EASIER, IT'S BEST TO "CLEAN BULK" WHEN YOU'RE MASS TRAINING. SOME PEOPLE DON'T CARE MUCH OUTSIDE OF GETTING THE RIGHT PROTEIN AND EAT EXCESSIVELY WHEN BULKING (DIRTY BULKING), WHICH MEANS THEY GAIN MORE FAT AND HAVE MORE TO STRIP OFF IN THE CUTTING PHASE. BIGGER BROTHER THINKS IT'S OK TO BE A BIT LENIENT WHEN BULKING, BUT DON'T MAKE YOUR LIFE MORE DIFFICULT BY CONSUMING LOTS OF UNNECESSARY CALORIES. THEN, WHEN YOU'RE CUTTING, YOU ONLY HAVE TO GO A COUPLE OF BODY FAT PERCENTAGE POINTS DOWN, WHICH IS EASIER AND LESS TAXING ON THE BODY. INTERESTINGLY, ARNOLD SCHWARZENEGGER ALWAYS STAYED WITHIN 10-15LBS (4-6KG) OF HIS COMPETITION WEIGHT, OFF-SEASON, WHILE FELLOW MULTIPLE MR. OLYMPIA, DORIAN YATES, WOULD VARY BY OVER 40LBS (18KGS)! AGAIN, THESE ARE EXTREME EXAMPLES, BUT YOU GET THE POINT.

For a lot of men, the cutting phase can be particularly frustrating as it ultimately involves losing weight, and size. The key thing is to minimise the loss of muscle, but it's tricky to get the balance. It's also important to remember, though, leaner bodies can look bigger, as the muscle is more defined, and it's not about weight as much as a balance in overall strength, fitness, look and symmetry. To minimise this, as a rule of thumb, when bulking you want to go bigger than your lean target so that when you cut, you settle leaner around the size you want.

When training in the cutting phase the simplest method can be to just shift towards strength endurance training by reducing the weight you would do in mass training and increase reps to a higher range, cut your rest time between sets to 30-45 seconds and add in extra interval training cardio (start with 1 x 30 minute session and then add in another session after 1-2 weeks). In terms of the training, just bear in mind that in this approach you want it to be intense and work your muscles hard, but you are not going for excessive muscle breakdown, as in mass training. Depending on how experienced you are with resistance training, you should be able to feel the point of excess. Work the muscles just to the point where you will notice they were trained the next day or so, but be aware they shouldn't be excessively sore with severe DOMS.

If you generally eat well, this change alone, with a minor reduction in calories, can make a big difference and in the case of people who are more naturally lean, it can get you very close to where you want to be without excessive dieting. If you tend towards the endomorphic body type, you may need to add in additional cardio, increase reps and be more careful with your nutrition.

Another simple method (if you are generally doing over six reps per set) is to continue your training as you are, but cut your rest times between sets to 45–60 seconds max. Keep the weight level as close to what you have been doing as possible, although you may need to drop the weight to complete the reps. Start with your usual weight, then drop down to keep the reps up. If you're a hard gainer you may want to keep the reps under 10, while endomorphs may want to go up to 12, or possibly even 20. It's always worth experimenting with rep ranges to see how your body responds. Try to complete your workout at a fast (controlled) pace. Similar to the above, finish your workout at a point where the muscles have been worked intensely, but won't suffer excessive DOMS for days. Alongside this, add in extra interval training cardio per week (start with 1 or 2 x 30 minute sessions and then add in another session after 1–2 weeks).

MAINTENANCE MODE

Maintenance mode is what Bigger Brother would describe as the balanced platform you are looking to build for yourself. It's that zone where you are comfortably and noticeably fit and healthy. It's not where you're ready to compete with a top fitness model with sub 10% body fat, but can be very close. Think sporty, athletic movie hero! It's a comfortable level, where you won't feel starved of energy, but will appear lean and fitter than the majority of people. The reason it's a "platform" is because it will allow you to balance your everyday fitness and give you the benefits of that fitness across other aspects of your life, from confidence to better work performance and more energy. It will allow you some indulgence with limited impact, if that is what you want, but it's also an effective platform to more easily build into an even more advanced physique or train for a new physical challenge more rapidly. That might be anything from Ironman to Spartan Race, or even a short few weeks to be camera-ready for a Men's Health magazine cover.

For most people, particularly those in busy, sedentary jobs and with a work commute that means it's hard to find time for exercise, reaching maintenance mode is a great way to balance life and other career aspirations. One of the things Bigger Brother sees most often is people leaping in with an overly pumped mindset, so common in the period just after Christmas. The media and fitness advertising is telling you it's your time, you can be indestructible in a matter of days. The New Year resolution kicks in after the December binge, you sign up for Tough Mudder in three months, buy all the latest gear, plan your new pumping playlist on Spotify, drop eating down to salads and buy a few fancy protein shakes. You go for it hard, with great intentions, but an approach that isn't thought through (or right for you) can hit the body (and mind) hard, sending it crashing and burning in a matter of weeks as the lack of results, other life impacts and energy drain kills the motivation.

This boom and bust approach is all too common and, although it starts with the right intentions, it doesn't usually deliver long-term results. Generally, what works best is preparation, focus and a steady, consistent approach that drives ongoing progress. That's not to say you shouldn't push the body with intense exercise, it's just that it needs to be done in the right way, with the right tools, knowledge and approach. Most people, even if overweight, can drop 10kg (22lbs) or more of fat and get to a reasonable maintenance mode quicker than they might think, even if they haven't been exercising. The body is an amazing thing; it adapts relatively quickly if you treat it the right way and move at the right pace for you.

A NOTE ABOUT EATING:

IT'S OFTEN THOUGHT OR PERCEIVED IN GENERAL SOCIETY THAT GAINING FAT (OR GENERAL "WEIGHT", AS IT'S SO OFTEN REFERRED TO) IS FASTER AND EASIER THAN LOSING FAT. IN PRINCIPLE, THERE IS NO REAL DIFFERENCE IN SPEED. IT'S ONLY THAT IT'S EASIER IN THE WORLD WE LIVE IN TO EAT FATTY, SUGARY, CALORIE-DENSE FOODS, AS THEY ARE SO READILY AVAILABLE AND SEEM TO TASTE SO GREAT. I'M NO SCIENTIST, BUT IT'S PROBABLY NO ACCIDENT THAT THESE

CALORIE DENSE FOODS APPEAL TO US. ONCE UPON A TIME, WE PROBABLY NEEDED TO EAT MORE FATTY FOODS SO THEY COULD BE STORED IN THE BODY TO SURVIVE – AS THE NEXT ROUND OF QUALITY FOOD WAS ONLY AVAILABLE WHEN ONE OF THE HUNTERS MANAGED TO KILL THE NEXT WILD DEER WITH HIS STONE AND STICK SPEAR. OUR MINDS AND ENVIRONMENT SEEM TO HAVE EVOLVED MUCH QUICKER THAN OUR BODIES' TASTE FOR FOOD, SO NOW THAT IT'S READILY AVAILABLE, IT'S EASY TO BE DRAWN TO IT. THEY SAY BOOZE – OR MORE, THE EFFECT OF ALCOHOL ON THE BRAIN – ROLLS US BACK TO OUR MORE PRIMAL MINDSET. PERHAPS THAT'S WHY WE ARE SO OFTEN DRIVEN TO STUFF KEBABS, BURGERS AND ALL MANNER OF OTHER DIRTY FOOD INTO OUR BODIES WHEN INTOXICATED!

FORTUNATELY, IT TAKES SURPRISINGLY LESS TIME THAN YOU MIGHT THINK TO CHANGE THE WAY YOUR BODY (AND MIND) TREATS FOOD. I CAN'T SAY IT'S EASY TO GET THERE, AND IT ULTIMATELY DEPENDS ON YOU HOW LONG IT TAKES, BUT I CAN SAY THAT IT DOES GET EASIER AS YOU GET CLOSER TO MAINTENANCE MODE.

Over the years, the author and his Bigger Brother have been lucky enough to be complimented on their physiques from time to time. On certain occasions, there have been some quite bizarre backhanded compliments from random people, accusing us of using steroids or having the "right genetics". That's something we find quite amusing, as it's not the truth! The main point here is, once you are in or on your way to maintenance mode, people take notice. Sadly, possibly due to the human condition, it's often perceived as lucky, down to some sort of secret, endless hours in a gym or through cheating, rather than knowledge, experience and the right focused effort. By reading this book you will already be way ahead of the majority; you just have to apply it and go for it!

As highlighted earlier in this book, there is no secret – neither my Bigger Brother nor I have particularly great genetics for fitness, strength or muscle development, and we don't do super-strict complex diets or secret gym techniques. However, we've reached a point where, with a combination of (Bigger Brother) knowledge and experience, we can maintain with as little as three hours of training a week and without strict dieting. Now, this doesn't mean our training is low intensity, we don't do any work and we don't think about eating, but we are able to balance lean, athletic physiques alongside full-time jobs while enjoying some fun food (and drink) as well.

When I say this, I'm not saying we aim to maintain 6–10% body fat magazine-cover-ready bodies all year round, eat what we want and just get stronger and stronger. Bear in mind that the camera can add 10lbs (4.5kg), so being that lean can actually make you look gaunt in the face – off-camera. The reality is that level isn't easily achieved 100% of the time for most people (certainly not for non-professional athlete or model, or those that are not genetically gifted) without stepping up a gear in some form and throwing in some regular intense cardio and stricter nutrition.

The goal is to stay within a couple of kilograms – essentially, within 1-3 weeks (depending on how quickly your body adapts) – of that level so that by stepping up cardio and adjusting your diet you can do short cut or bulking periods. So even if you don't want to be a fitness model or bodybuilder, if a magazine ever calls you, then you can be ready quickly! ;)

NOTE: BIGGER BROTHER FINDS IT QUITE INTERESTING WHEN READING OR HEARING ARNOLD SCHWARZENEGGER TALK ABOUT HOW IMPORTANT POSING AND "DISPLAY" WAS/IS TO HIS WINS AND WINNING A COMPETITION. WHILE THIS BOOK IS NOT ABOUT BEING A PRO BODY ATHLETE AS SUCH, IT'S INTERESTING, BECAUSE THE MEDIA OFTEN SUGGESTS OR LEADS PEOPLE TO BELIEVE THAT BODIES CAN BE "PERFECT". IN HIS BOOKS AND INTERVIEWS, ARNOLD HAS TALKED ABOUT SLOPING SHOULDERS AND AVOIDING COMPETING DIRECTLY WITH A COMPETITOR WHO MIGHT HAVE A SUPERIOR BODY PART. THE POINT HERE IS THAT EVEN PROFESSIONALS HAVE WEAKER POINTS, AND DISPLAY OF THE BODY – WHETHER THAT INCLUDES POSITIONING, POSING, TAN/SKIN COLOUR, CLOTH-ING, LIGHTING, QUALITY OF PHOTOGRAPHY, THROUGH TO USE OF PHOTOSHOP ENHANCEMENTS – CAN PLAY A PART IN THE IMAGES WE ARE BOMBARDED WITH IN THE MEDIA. SO, DON'T

BE TOO HARD ON YOURSELF. IT'S OK TO STRIVE FOR PER-FECTION BUT BEAR IN MIND NOTHING IS EVER COMPLETELY PERFECT (CERTAINLY NOT ALL OF THE TIME) AND FINAL PRESENTATION MAKES A DIFFERENCE.

This type of maintenance is based on being at the size and shape you want, so that as long as you do the right things with your training and diet most of the time (over 80%), a couple of less healthy meals a week can be countered with a dial up in your training or a healthy, low calorie compensation at another meal. This can also include alcohol and, while drinking doesn't really help progress, if you're an adult and enjoy a beer or two (as we do) it doesn't have to be completely off the cards.

A NOTE ON BOOZE:

WHEN DRINKING, YOU SHOULD CONSIDER AVOIDING ALL OUT BINGES (PARTICULARLY FOLLOWING HEAVY GYM SESSIONS) AND ENSURE YOU HAVE GIVEN YOUR BODY THE APPROPRIATE NUTRITION WITHIN YOUR CALORIE LEVEL. A FEW BEERS COM-PENSATED FOR BY SOME GOOD MEALS ON THE DAY, WITHIN THE LEEWAY OF CALORIE INTAKE, AND SOME COMPENSATION CARDIO/TRAINING THE DAY BEFORE OR AFTER, WILL ENSURE YOU CAN ENJOY SOME SINS. IT ALSO KEEPS YOU SANE! THIS QUOTE (WHICH CAN BE FOUND WITH A SEARCH ONLINE) FROM ACTOR, JASON MOMOA, SAYS IT ALL!

YOU NEED TO EAT BIG AND LIFT BIG. BUT I PREFER TO EAT AS MUCH LEAN MEAT AND GREEN VEG AS POSSIBLE AND SAVE THE CALORIES FOR GUINNESS. IT KEEPS YOU SANE.

JASON MOMOA

The trick is consistency. Your body tends to reflect what you do the majority of the time. In the same way as you are unlikely to change your body composition with one gym session, one or two meals out of 20 won't change your composition instantly. Also, when you have some muscle mass and you've applied some consistency with your generally good diet, your body is going to have a faster metabolism and be better at staying lean. The only caveat is that if you are in the low levels of body fat (under 10%) and topless, it can be more noticeable that you just ate a big burger, but that is only temporary. Not to mention your body will probably still look way better than most on the beach! Actually, as long as you are getting the nutrients in your diet to feed your training, the limited variations in calories with "cheat meals" and/or "cheat drinking" during the week can even help keep your metabolism moving, as long as your average intake of calories across the week is not regularly overshooting your level of physical activity.

Bigger Brother thinks that part of the problem people find with reaching their goals and maintaining improvements through exercise and diet is due to the media sending out mixed messages and varied advice. People yo-yo around with training and diet, force themselves not to eat or drink certain things for set periods, put themselves into crazed states by over-restricting things, then they binge when they finish – and it's human nature to want things you can't have or haven't had! The reality is, it's easier to control your desires for short periods then give yourself small rewards (before cravings turn into out of control desires to binge). Bit by bit, and step by step you will eventually reach the summit. As long as you can make the short periods add up to "most of the time", you will start to get the consistency needed for maintenance. The great thing is, by not restricting yourself completely, you start to enjoy the things that are good for you, you get more pleasure out of the times you have the bad, but you find yourself naturally preferring the things that are good for you most of the time.

Tips For Maintenance

☑ Keep your good habits up at least 75-80% of the time (ideally 80%+). Think of it as a consistency scale of 0-100%, with each -10% increment equalling the 1-2 week period of additional training and strict diet to get to your current 100%

(or really your 97%, as there is always room for improvement!). Although note that if you start dropping below 80%, and particularly 70%, the extra work required exponentially increases.

☑ During maintenance you don't have to consistently push your body to failure, as you do when building mass. It's important to train intensely, but listen to your body. Take it to the point where you feel you have sufficiently hit the body parts you are exercising hard, but not to the point where it's likely to give you soreness (DOMS) for days. This is easier than it sounds, when your muscles are reasonably well trained, as it will take you more to push the muscles beyond their current level, plus at a greater level of awareness of your body, you know when your training will hit you hardest.

☑ Ensure you know your ideal average calorie intake for your size and compensate any cheat meals with some cardio and good meals. While calorie counting isn't always necessary, it's good to get familiar with the ball park levels and what calories you're actually-eating, so you can keep on top of it without too much effort day to day. Check out the macronutrients calculator on The Lean Exec website:
BIT.LY/TLE-MACROCAL

☑ Do power exercises, like deadlifts and squats, once per week. Use a weight where you can lift 10 reps a set and cut rest times between sets to under 1 minute 15 seconds.

☑ It's useful to experiment with eating in the evening to see how it affects your body. Everyone is different, so while some people swear by no carbs in the evening, others don't see a major difference, so long as their average macronutrients and calorie levels during the day are OK for their size and physical activity.

☑ Eat three good healthy meals during the day and ensure you eat healthy snacks regularly – before you get hungry – to avoid cravings and bingeing. A good rule of thumb is not to go for more than about 3–4 hours without eating something nourishing. This can be as simple as a handful of nuts or some milk.

NOTE: SOME PEOPLE PREFER TO EAT 5–6 SMALL MEALS A DAY, BUT THIS CAN SOMETIMES BE DIFFICULT, DEPENDING ON WORK OR STUDY COMMITMENTS. SMALL, HEALTHY SNACKS OR A PROTEIN SHAKE BETWEEN MAIN MEALS CAN BE AN EASIER WAY TO MANAGE THIS WITHOUT IMPACTING YOUR LIFE SCHEDULE.

TEMPO & TENSION IN RESISTANCE TRAINING

As mentioned at various points in this book, having advanced muscles is ultimately helpful in knowing when the muscles are being trained effectively. The reality is, like all other components of training, your body starts to adapt so, ultimately, you need to vary your tempo and tension to optimise your results. The more experienced you are, the more likely you are to know what you need to do to achieve this.

The challenge for people who are less familiar with resistance training, and particularly beginners, is they can't always assess accurately whether they are training the muscles the right way. At the very beginning, or after periods when you have not trained for a long time, it's relatively easy to create intensity and overload the muscle, as pretty much everything you do at this stage is overload. However, while generally speaking the most effective way to increase progressive overload is to add more weight, once the muscles "catch up", and the more you advance, the more you may need to find ways to "surprise" your muscles.

This is why beginners will often be enthusiastic for the first few weeks, while they see very quick results. However, they lose motivation as their methods start to lose momentum and hypertrophy is required for progress. This is where the rep speed (tempo) and time under tension may need more attention.

Rep Speed; The Basics

Most books on training and bodybuilding mention the speed of reps, which is usually referred to as the "tempo". Essentially, tempo is the speed at which you lift, push, pull or hold the weight at various points through an exercise repetition.

Different parts of the repetition:

☑ The concentric part of a rep is typically when the muscle is being engaged and shortened under tension.

☑ The eccentric part of the rep is typically when the muscle is being engaged and lengthened under tension.

☑ Depending on the body part you are training, the concentric or eccentric points can be at different points in the repetition. For example, in a bicep curl, the concentric part of the movement is the first part, when you curl the weight up, shortening and squeezing the bicep. While doing a triceps push-down, the part where the arm is bending is eccentric, as the triceps muscle is being stretched, with the concentric part happening as you push down.

Why is repetition speed important? Well, the main reason is it can have different effects, but also if your body/muscles do the same thing over and over again they adapt and just get used to the movement, making it less effective. In principle, if the reps are faster, the time under tension is lower. If you do the same motion with a more controlled, slower movement, the tension of each rep is higher, although it's worth noting that the weight and number of reps are also important. Arguably, if you did double the number of reps at double the speed, the time under tension would be the same overall.

This is why you have to listen to your body and learn to understand how it responds. Think of it like muscle meditation. Essentially, high muscle tension plus progressive overload equals muscle progress (assuming rest and nutrition). However, to varying degrees, different speed and tension techniques will work at different times for different people.

If you're starting out, or perhaps haven't been thinking enough about the speed at which you are performing movements, a reasonable aim is:

☑ One second during the concentric, positive motion (muscle shortening).

☑ Slightly slower at two to three seconds, when lowering the weight in the eccentric, negative motion (muscle lengthening).

Ultimately, though, the most important thing is to raise and lower a weight with control, no matter what the speed, and try to concentrate and learn how the movement is affecting your muscle. Does it feel tight? Can you squeeze the specific muscle at the top or stretch the muscle at the bottom? Monitoring this will help you become more in tune with your body and how it responds.

Thinking About Tempo In A More Advanced Way

It's easy to look at rep speed as simply the time to raise and lower the weight. However, keep in mind a pause at the top and or bottom. As an example, let's look at a common movement like the bench press:

Step	Movement	Rep
1	Lift the bar off the rack	
2	Lower the weight to your chest (eccentric chest contraction)	2 seconds
3	Stretch the chest at the bottom position	1 second
4	Raise the weight (concentric chest contraction)	2 seconds
5	Squeeze the chest in the contracted top position	1 second

IMPORTANT:

IN TRAINING PLANS, THIS TEMPO STRUCTURE IS REPRESENTED AS FOUR NUMBERS: 2121

Experimenting with different times at each stage of the movement will help you to discover how tension works on your muscles for each movement. Just ensure that whatever you do, the movement is controlled and you are lifting safely (e.g. safety bars and/or a spotter).

Tempo & Tension For Different Exercises

Speed of reps and time under tension isn't a new concept and has been around in bodybuilding and strength training for many years. However, in the midst of a workout, particularly when gym time is limited, it's easy to forget about this, and also about stretching and squeezing muscles. In addition, we might forget the key differences there can be with different exercises.

If you want to ensure you're getting the best bang for your buck out of each exercise, then it's important to think about the exercise and where you are applying time. In other words, there are different points in each exercise movement where tension is high and low. For example, in the case of a squat, there is the least amount of tension when you are standing, whereas tension is highest as you lower into the squat position. For bicep curls, when at the top or bottom of the movement there is limited tension, but the tension increases rapidly as soon as you start to drop or raise the dumbbells, so making use of the bicep.

While some people might say there is no benefit to holding at an "off tension" position, Bigger Brother would say there are some benefits. For example, in the last reps of the set, particularly towards the end of a workout, when it's getting tough and you might need a moment or two to gather your physical (and mental) strength to complete the reps. This can be particularly useful on big movements, like squats, where it can require a lot of willpower to push out the final few reps.

NOTE: MILK SQUATS! THIS IS AN OLD-SCHOOL BODYBUILDING TECHNIQUE FOR BUILDING LEG MUSCLE, BUT ALSO THE ENTIRE BODY. THIS IS WHERE YOU DO HEAVY (AND CONTROLLED) SQUATS FOR 20 REPS. DUE TO THE HIGHER VOLUME, AND PARTICULARLY TOWARDS THE END OF THE SET, YOU ARE LIKELY TO NEED TO REST A LITTLE LONGER IN THE STANDING POSITION. THIS MIGHT ONLY BE A COUPLE OF SECONDS, BUT ENOUGH TO GATHER THE FOCUS TO COMPLETE THE NEXT REP. I THINK THEY THEN DRANK LOTS OF MILK AS PART OF THE RECOVERY, WHICH IS WHY THEY CALL THEM MILK SQUATS. IT WOULD SEEM TO MAKE SENSE, AS BOTH ARNOLD SCHWARZENEGGER AND HIS AUSTRALIAN REINCARNATION, CALUM VON MOGER, BOTH PUBLICLY MENTION THE IMPORTANCE OF SQUATTING AND MILK IN THEIR MUSCLE GROWTH.

The key thing to be mindful of is stretching/squeezing points and where the movement is most difficult. For some movements, the tension decreases in the contracted (positive) position, typically pushing movements or movements where the arms or legs lock out, like bench press, shoulder press, squatting, leg pressing, etc.

So, when you are in this position, it's doing less for your muscles. The really important point in these exercises is going to be the eccentric or negative position, where the muscle is "stretched", and this is a point where holding for a few seconds could be useful.

For example:

Bench (or dumbbell) press: there is an opportunity to stretch the chest in the lower position. The tension will be lower when the arms are straight, as it's not just your muscles supporting the weight. As you lower the weight to your chest, tension on the muscles will increase. It's worth noting, though, that for chest movements you should aim to "squeeze" the chest together in the contracted, positive position.

With other exercises, like bicep curls, leg curls, seated rows, and lateral raises, you're looking for the squeeze, as these exercises have less tension in the eccentric (negative) position and more tension at or near the contracted (positive) position. The ideal point to hold for a few seconds is going to be when the muscle is being "squeezed" and tensed.

For example:

Bicep curls: there is an opportunity to squeeze the muscle when raised in the positive contracted position at the top of the movement. It should be a tight feeling in the bicep as it holds the weight in position. However, it's also important to note that to some degree your bones are supporting this position so the points where your arms are neither fully straight nor bent will be those with the highest tension. The lower the weight, the more it will put tension on your lower bicep, then shifting to the top of your bicep as you raise the weight. This is very similar to leg curls.

While most exercises tend to lean towards a dominant positive or negative tension point, some exercises allow for both. This is particularly relevant to calf training, where standing and seated calf raises allow for a stretch and hold at the top and bottom of the movement. Lat pulldowns are another example where a tension stretch and squeeze can be achieved at both points in the movement.

As mentioned above, there will be no standard rep speed/tempo to use for the rest of your training life. Variation will be important for rounded development and improvement, so don't worry if this seems like a lot to remember. The most important thing is to practise feeling the difference between each point in a movement and how the speed impacts that feeling. The more you do it, the more natural it becomes, and you are likely to begin enjoying the tense feeling, which is essentially your muscles filling with blood.

WARMING UP, STRETCHING & COOLING DOWN

As any fitness professional or personal trainer will tell you, warming up, stretching and cooling down are important elements of your training. There are certain common ways and recommendations for how to do these, which are highlighted below.

WARMING UP

Warming up is typically done with cardio exercises, e.g. running, using the cross trainer (elliptical), rowing, jumping rope, etc. The typical recommended approach would be that a warm up should be done at around 45–55% of your maximum capacity or, in other words, a fast-paced walk or light jog for between 5–10 mins. The science says that depending on size and fitness, most people will warm up sometime after 5 and before 10 mins. You'll know your body is warmed up when your cheeks feel warm (note: that's your face cheeks, not your bum cheeks!).

The commonly referenced reasons for warming up are increasing blood flow, and loosening muscles and joints. While this is not untrue, what a simple search online will show you is that the newest research suggests it's more than that. Warming up effectively kicks your cellular energy systems into gear. Adenosine triphosphate (ATP) is what the body uses to transport energy within cells and even just a 1-2 degree increase in body temperature is significant enough to increase the rate of ATP breakdown. This is good, because the faster your ATP molecules break down, the more energy will be available for the body and this, in turn, increases nerve conduction and muscle contraction velocity. In other words, this should make you more ready to train, have more energy, and loosen up the muscles and tendons, which will help you to avoid injury.

There are also more descriptive methods of defining "being warmed up" and these include feeling warm over your whole body, feeling more loose/less tense, light sweating and an increase in breathing rate. In addition, there is some research that suggests some people need up to 30 mins to get warmed up! Based on some people I see in the gym, I think that might even be three hours! :)

In any case, you need to figure out what works for you. My approach has always been to do 5-10 minutes of running (ideally to the gym, not on a treadmill). Start slow, at around 40% capacity, or a gentle jog, and elevate to around 65-70% in the last minute or so. I go a bit faster than the bog-standard recommended, but never to a level that will mean I'm tired going into my training. The Bigger Brother thought here is that starting sessions is the hardest part. Elevating to a reasonable level will release some endorphins and get you over the hump. It's better to go into the session feeling alive and pumped than still lacklustre. Listen to your body, try to push yourself, but don't overdo it. Focus on building, not busting!

DYNAMIC STRETCHING

If you don't know already, dynamic stretching is essentially moving while you stretch. It's become very popular in sport and advocates will highlight its importance for loosening up muscles and joints, activating muscles, and improving the range of motion, as well as improving muscular performance. Based on some of the exercise positions, they are likely to help balance and co-ordination as well. The Lean Exec approach prescribed by Bigger Brother in this book doesn't include dynamic stretch routines, mainly because we are focused on efficiency of effort. The ideal is that if you have done the groundwork, as shown in the book, start your session with the cardio warm up, as suggested, do body weight or a light first set of movements (with full range of motion), and stretch muscles prior to sets and during rest periods, you are essentially doing a form of dynamic stretching. However, if you are a beginner, very unfit, have a concern about joint, ligament or muscle issues and/or anything else for that matter, you should consider trying some dynamic stretching or at least some more traditional stretching routines. You can find some of these resources on The Lean Exec website:

BIT.LY/TLE-STRETCH

COOLING DOWN (WARMING DOWN)

Cooling or warming down is essentially the opposite of a warm up, where the intensity decreases to a slow pace at the end of a training session. For the purposes of core Lean Exec training, cooling down is integrated into the cardio at the end of a workout, although you could choose to do this separately. In principle, it's good practice to finish a session by dropping the pace of your activity to low intensity in the last 2–5 or even 10 minutes. This could be as simple as dropping a run down to a jog and then walking for a couple of minutes before stopping. You could also do some static stretching, which has been said to reduce soreness, although Bigger Brother thinks a cold (ideally ice) bath is more effective! Whatever the case, try not to stop your training too suddenly – give yourself a few minutes to lower the intensity and reduce down to a more normal resting state. This also helps to avoid exercise blood pooling where blood and waste products like lactic acid remain in the muscles causing pain and swelling.

REST & REST DURATION

When talking about fitness, a lot of focus is put on being active, training and diet. While these are all very important, without appropriate rest and consideration of rest duration, your training can be less effective and even have negative results. The funny thing is, what's required in the gym takes up a smaller proportion of time than rest (and nutrition) and it's amazing how many people don't consider their time spent resting both inside and outside the gym.

Rest In The Gym

When I go to the gym, I don't carry much other than a towel, but I wear a Casio with a stopwatch. After I finish a set, I hit the start button on the watch and track my rest time. When the numbers hit my desired rest time, I hit the stop button, pick up the weights and do another set. While the time frame can vary depending on my goals at the time, this is consistent. On the days when I forget my watch I count out the seconds in my head, although I rarely forget my watch!

This is one of the most important habits for my training. The reason is that varying degrees of intensity are important, not just in terms of lifting different weights, but also in all aspects of the workout in relation to goals. While I have extensive understanding of my body's response to training and can gauge reasonably well how much time I need between sets without timing specifically, it's a good way to stay focused and avoid sloppy workouts.

Every time I go to the gym I see people sitting around, looking at their phones, talking on their phones, chatting to people, etc., between their sets. Not only are they usually resting way too long, they're also not focused on what they're doing. On the other hand, I see people doing endless reps and sets with little rest in between. I also notice that some of these people can be in the gym when I arrive and still there when I leave, 45-60 minutes later! While I don't know the details of their lives, nutrition or their progress, you do start to see certain patterns. They become lacklustre in their training, don't noticeably progress (or progress very slowly), get an injury, start using a PT or disappear from the gym altogether.

Unfortunately, the above mentioned relates to a couple of paradigms that persist in "fitness society". One is laziness (or, perhaps more accurately, lack of focus) and the other is "more is better". Bigger Brother knows that "time" spent in a gym or doing exercise is not directly related to progress! How you feel (fitness) and how you look in a mirror are more important in many ways than what the weighing scales say, and in a similar way, intensity in physical training often corresponds better to results than time. Time is important, but so is avoiding overtraining. Short, intense, frequent sessions can be far more effective than long, drawn out sessions. In other words, in terms of time in the gym, for most people (not including professionals/athletes) keep your gym sessions under one hour. This is more than enough time (a session) to do the work required for a great physique. Actually, longer sessions can be detrimental and cause muscle breakdown, not to mention overtraining. In addition, and if you want some science, cortisol levels naturally increase during training which, in turn, increases blood sugar levels and the body's ability to fight inflammation. This can be helpful, but excessive cortisol release can reduce the body's ability to use protein effectively, as well as inhibit muscle growth. Avoiding this is most easily done by keeping sessions short, not to mention short sessions mean more time for other things in life!

In terms of rest duration during training, while individuals will find certain time frames work best for them, there are some general ranges to stick to for good results. If you experiment with different times within the ranges you will soon find your sweet spot.

Reps & Rest In The Gym Guide

Training For Strength & Muscle Gains

Reps	Weight Range % 1 Rep Max	Rest Between Sets Seconds	Notes
1–4	90–100	75–300	For most people under 120 seconds (2 minutes) will work well, with the main difference coming down to your body type. If you're more ectomorphic, you may want to experiment with longer rest times when lifting for 1–2 reps – e.g. 3–5 minutes (although try to keep it under 3 minutes). If you're endomorphic, you may want to avoid going over 2 minutes.
5–8	80–90	60–120	While it's almost impossible to have a one-size-fits-all model, working in this range can deliver results for most people, unless your body leans very ectomorphic or endomorphic.
9–12	70–80	45–120	This range is not recommended for people who are more ectomorphic beginners or find gaining strength and size more difficult. It may do no long-term harm to experiment in this range, but if your goal is to increase strength and size, Bigger Brother recommends working in lower rep ranges.

Generally speaking, regardless of your body type, if your goal is size and strength, working under 8 reps is likely to have faster results. Bigger Brother generally suggests starting (after warm up) with higher weight (75%+ of one rep max), under six reps and rest around two minutes for pushing past plateaus and increasing strength. Once you have reached a size a few kilograms beyond your ideal lean muscle size, increasing reps and dropping rest time will become more useful.

NOTE: REMEMBER, IT'S GOOD TO FOCUS ON INCREASING YOUR STRENGTH FIRST – AS THIS WILL NATURALLY BUILD SIZE IF YOU ARE EATING CORRECTLY – THEN FOCUSING ON FURTHER MUSCLE DEFINITION, IF THAT'S WHAT YOU WANT. AS MENTIONED IN OTHER SECTIONS OF THIS BOOK, PART OF THE REASON PRO BODYBUILDERS WORK IN HIGH REP RANGES IS BECAUSE THEY CAN ALREADY LIFT SERIOUS WEIGHT! MUCH OF WHAT THEY ARE DOING IS CONDITIONING WITH HEAVY WEIGHT. SO, WORK YOUR WAY UP TO LIFTING HEAVY, THEN YOU CAN DO HIGHER REP CONDITIONING WORK FOR THAT STRONG MUSCULAR BODY YOU'VE DEVELOPED!

Reps & Rest In The Gym Guide

Training For Lean

Reps	Weight Range % 1 Rep Max	Rest Between Sets Seconds	Notes
5–8	75–85%	45–120	This range is likely to work better for people who are more ectomorphic.
9–12	65–75%	45–90	This range can work for a lot of people when cutting, but be mindful of your body response and consider dropping or increasing weight and reps in correspondence with your body type lean.
12+	50–60%	30–60	This range is likely to work better for people who are more endomorphic, although some sessions working in higher rep ranges can work for all in this phase, as the goal is strength, endurance and a good pump, without excessive soreness.

Rest Outside Of The Gym

There seems to be an automatic mentality in society that going to a gym, doing exercise, and lifting weights directly equals better health, performance and/or improved muscle and fitness. To a degree this is true – going to a gym and doing some exercise is probably better than doing nothing, in most cases. However, doing it wrong and/or overdoing it can sometimes do more harm than good. Rest outside of the gym is as important as the other things you do outside of the gym, like eating.

Bigger Brother has found that intense training for shorter periods (as discussed above) coupled with sticking to a good weekly training plan that fits your lifestyle is one of the simplest ways to avoid overtraining. Another is more intuitive and can require some experience and knowledge of your own body's response to training. Essentially, a sense of how your body "feels" during and in the periods after training, which is something that develops the more you train. Depending on things, including your level of fitness, level of exertion, how much physical activity you do in your regular daily life, age, your body type and, more specifically, your body's unique ability to recover in the context of your daily life, means that rest needed varies for different people. There can sometimes be quite a thin line between intense training and overtraining, so it's important to manage this with appropriate rest between sessions.

In relation to the above, it's also important to remember that being mindful of rest doesn't mean you should avoid training just because you feel a bit tired or can't be bothered. The reality is, if you are training to advance your fitness and weight training, it's normal to have some soreness, tiredness and even (particularly if you are in you're 30+ and definitely 40+) to have some niggling aches here and there, although these effects should not be excessive and you shouldn't ignore real pain, as this can result in serious injury. They should feel good (in a strange way) as if you are content in having achieved something. Our bodies are designed to be used for physical activity but, unfortunately, modern life tends to put us in a position where it's easy to be lazy.

When this tendency is first being broken it can feel difficult, but after a while the body craves this feeling, a sort of "physical satisfaction" and thankfulness that it's being used. The resulting fitness can have fantastic effects as, in the same way that a strong mind can help create a strong body, a strong body can help create confidence and a strong mind. So, the ideal point of these minor effects, if your training, nutrition and rest are complementing each other correctly, is enough that you feel that your body is being worked hard and progressing, but it should not be at a level where it has a negative impact on your day-to-day life (the effect should be generally positive).

A NOTE FOR BEGINNERS (AND PEOPLE JUST GETTING BACK INTO TRAINING AFTER A LONG BREAK, ESPECIALLY THOSE IN THEIR 30S AND OLDER): THE REALITY IS THAT IF YOU ARE NOT USED TO TRAINING OR HAVE NOT TRAINED FOR A WHILE, THE FIRST ONE TO THREE MONTHS (POSSIBLY LONGER) CAN BE A CHALLENGE, DEPENDING ON YOUR FITNESS. THIS IS MAINLY BECAUSE UNTIL YOUR BODY IS CONDITIONED TO, OR BACK TO, A REASONABLE LEVEL, IT CAN HIT QUITE HARD. THIS IS WHERE THE POWER OF YOUR MIND AND YOUR WILLPOWER TO CHANGE HABITS IN YOUR LIFE WILL BE VERY IMPORTANT. YOU ARE MOST LIKELY GOING TO HAVE TO MAKE SOME ADJUSTMENTS TO MANAGE THIS, ALTHOUGH ONCE YOU GET PAST THIS HURDLE, IT DOES GET EASIER. THE MORE YOU TAKE CONTROL OF YOUR FITNESS, REST AND NUTRITION, THE QUICKER YOU CAN GET PAST THIS POINT WHERE MOST PEOPLE STOP. PRACTICE TRAINING YOUR MIND AND FOCUS ON PROGRESS IN STEPS; IT'S NOT A RACE, BUT RATHER A JOURNEY TO SOMETHING BETTER. REMEMBER, THERE CAN BE MANY REASONS FOR TRAINING AND IT'S GOOD TO SET A GOAL WITH AN EVENT OF SOME KIND, BUT THE MOST IMPORTANT ONE IS: "TRAINING FOR LIFE".

So, what is the right level of rest outside of the gym? Unfortunately, there is no exact answer, as everyone is different and each training session can be different, due to a number of factors. However, there are some general guidelines that you can follow until you know your body well enough to create your own bespoke schedule.

The following guidelines are based on three to five hours per week (e.g. three to five hours weight training sessions under one hour and one to three cardio sessions under a total of 60 minutes per week).

Description	Body Type			Notes
	Ecto	Meso	Endo	
Daily Sleep	Typically 7.5–9 hours			If you find it difficult to get more than 7 hours of sleep then short naps in the early afternoon may be a solution, if possible.
Heavy Lower Back Training Recovery	Up to one week			Assumes training has been sufficiently intense to cause DOMS.
Larger Muscle/Muscle Group Recovery (e.g. chest, back, upper legs, etc.)	48–72 hours	Around 48 hours	Min 48 hours	Assumes training has been sufficiently intense to cause DOMS.
Small Muscle/Muscle Group Recovery (e.g. biceps, triceps, etc.)	24–48 hours	24–36 hours	Min 24 hours	Assumes training has been sufficiently intense to cause DOMS.
Excessive DOMS	Avoid retraining the muscle until DOMS has peaked and has been subsiding.			This can be identified as a reduction in soreness to the point where the "dull" soreness is only felt by flexing or tightening the muscle.

Notes

☑ Active recovery with lower intensity training that increases blood flow can help to speed up the recovery process, although it's usually better to wait until the peak of DOMS has started to reduce before training a muscle specifically, i.e. if you have some excessive soreness for multiple days, some lighter exercising of the muscles one to three days later can help to ease and speed up recovery.

☑ All body types should see recovery times reduce to a degree as the body becomes more developed/"trained". However, major pushes in training progress to increase strength and growth of muscles may reduce less for those with more ectomorphic tendencies.

☑ The important thing is to learn to read your body and avoid (over) training a body part before it has had a chance to recover to a level at which it can perform equal to or better than the previous session. Training a muscle hard before it has recovered can have negative effects on strength, growth and performance. Muscle recovery is a key part of hypertrophy and general progress.

☑ If your goal is to gain strength and muscle and you are regularly experiencing excessive DOMS, you may find it necessary to experiment with a reduction in your cardio activities or increasing your cardio to see how this impacts your recovery and gaining progress. It's probably not helpful to do more than 60-90 mins of running in a week on top of training, but doing some regular cardio is likely to help your blood flow and your recovery.

☑ Extra sleep can help to speed up recovery. I think it's probably one of the most important factors. If you aren't getting enough sleep, it's harder to train, harder to recover and harder to improve. If you're a bad sleeper, like me, try the sleep suggestions in our sleep supplement on The Lean Exec website: BIT.LY/TLE-SLEEP

☑ Ensuring your nutrition and particularly macro calories are sufficient for your training is important to aid recovery (see Diet & Nutrition section).

DIET & NUTRITION

Training is, of course, important for stimulating your body in ways that will improve its ability to perform. However, like a machine, your body needs the right raw materials, energy and maintenance to perform at its optimum level. Understanding the importance of nutrition, what is quality fuel and how much your body needs, is as important as (some would say, more important than) what you do in training. The benefits of good nutrition also stretch beyond your training. Not only do they help recovery and rebuilding, they also improve the general health of your body, from your nervous system to your immune system, optimising your body, inside and out. Therefore, what you consume in your everyday "diet" is important to maximising your results.

However, I often think that the word "diet" is used by media and general society in a skewed way. There are two definitions of "diet" in the *Oxford English Dictionary*, but it tends to be the second that people fixate on.

DIET

/DʌɪəT/

1. The kinds of food that a person, animal, or community habitually eat, E.g. "a vegetarian diet"

SYNONYMS: *selection of food, food and drink, food, foodstuffs, provisions, edibles, fare*

2. A special course of food to which a person restricts themselves, either to lose weight or for medical reasons, E.g. "I'm going on a diet"

SYNONYMS: *dietary regime, dietary regimen, dietary programme, restricted diet, crash diet*

So much emphasis is put on the second definition, which is a very short-term view and plays to the yo-yo, boom and bust scenario described earlier in this book. It's always about playing catch up, looking for the fast solution, the quick fix, the difficult, restrictive approach that requires so much willpower, it feels like an achievement or insurmountable hurdle. Rather, Bigger Brother prefers to focus on the first definition, the food that is consistently consumed. No one gets fit and healthy just eating salad. While you might lose weight while restricting your food, it doesn't automatically mean that's good for you. Healthy, fit exercising bodies need consistent quality food and you'll find if you generally focus on eating an overall better diet rather than suddenly sprinting into a highly restrictive diet or going for hours on end without eating, your body is likely to respond better in the long run.

Actually, sudden restriction of calorie intake can have the opposite effect to the one desired; the body thinks it won't be getting fed for a while so starts to do what it does to survive – slow the metabolism and start storing fat up, in case the next meal is a while away. This issue is further enhanced when somebody comes off a strict diet and rapidly gains weight again, as the metabolism has slowed down, but the food intake has suddenly increased. There is science in this, but it is common sense. We live (at least in the First World countries) in a situation where food is relatively "available", but our bodies have not intrinsically changed from centuries ago, when food was not so easy to come by. The body has inbuilt ways of keeping us alive, even when we don't need it, so we have to "train" the body so it knows that it doesn't need to store excess, because the next meal is not far away. Despite this reality, for some reason the media and the world in general seems to perceive something different. It's true that calorie restriction can help you to lose weight, but sudden, short-term or sporadic calorie restriction is not usually the answer.

Training and what you do in the gym is important. However, without the right fuel in your body's engine you're likely to struggle to get the results you want (particularly as your body ages). In the same way that if you fill a car with the wrong fuel, it will run poorly and be less efficient, if you fill your body with the wrong food and substances, it is unlikely to perform at its best. Also like a car, if you use your body for longer, it will need more of the appropriate fuel to keep going.

The key starting point to good diet and nutrition is understanding what your particular body needs in relation to the amount/level of physical (and mental) exertion you are putting it through. While there are some key things that apply to most people, everything from our height, weight, the chemical reactions in our body, through to our personal goals can impact how we approach diet and nutrition.

The right balance of quality and quantity is important. In training, in particular, you are balancing the need to improve and/or grow strong muscle, while staying lean. This relies heavily on calories (quantity) and types of calories (quality). The most common mistakes people make when it comes to diet and training are finding and/or knowing the right balance in relation to their targets. Perhaps surprisingly, with training it's also common to find people who exercise and eat "healthy", but just don't realise they *aren't eating enough* to reap the full rewards of their training.

Generally speaking, most people are doing one of the following that is detrimental to their training progress:

☑ Eating and drinking way too many bad calories (the obvious one that gets all the headlines).

☑ Not consuming enough good calories for their training needs.

☑   Eating healthy foods, but not consuming the right calorie balance for their targets.

What many don't realise is that one bad calorie meal can equal 20–100% of their daily calories, while eating the same volume of good quality food might only represent 10–30%. So people think, "I'm not eating that much, as I only had two meals today," but in fact they are pushing 120%+ of their calorie requirement in two sittings! Not to mention they had 6–8 hours between meals, so their metabolism is receiving signals to slow down. On the other hand, people are eating lots of good food during the day, but only hitting 70% of their requirement. Both of these scenarios can be detrimental and they can both promote a slow metabolism.

In the first case, the person is likely going for hours without eating, and then gorging, which makes the body think it needs to store food for the long periods without food, and in the second case, the body is not getting enough to fuel its daily needs so, in response, holds onto what it can and even cannibalises muscle to find the fuel it needs. The chart below shows some examples of volume-to-calorie difference in healthy and unhealthy foods. Note the lower volume of less healthy food can be significantly more calories than a healthy source.

WEIGHT & CALORIES AS A PERCENTAGE (%) OF AVERAGE ADULT MALE DAILY CALORIE INTAKE*

Food Vs Food	Weight Grams	Calories Kcal	Of Daily %
Chicago Town Pizza (Pepperoni)	150	460	20%
VS			
2x Chicken Breast, Sweet Potato & Broccoli cooked with 10ml of Olive Oil	387	406	18%
VS			
2x Chicken Breast, Sweet Potato & Broccoli cooked with no Olive Oil	377	316	14%
VS			
Pret Chicken Salad with Dressing	237	547	24%
VS			
McDonald's Big Mac	216	590	26%
VS			
2x Chicken Breasts, Green Beans, Roast Potatoes, slice of Ham, Rice Pudding dessert	526	451	19%
VS			
KFC 2x Original Recipe Breasts, 1x Drumstick, side of Wedges	350	1050	45%
VS			
Milk Chocolate	40	410	18%
VS			
Greek Yogurt with 15g Honey	115	90	4%
VS			
Large Fish & Chips	849	1442	62%

*THE DAILY CALORIE INTAKE % ABOVE IS BASED ON THE MALE AVERAGE, WHICH IS USUALLY QUOTED AT 2,500 CALORIES PER DAY.

EXAMPLES OF LOW & HIGH QUALITY FOODS

So, you can probably see clearly the large difference it makes with even one bad calorie meal added to your diet in a day. In addition, and in principle, basic weight loss and weight gain can be boiled down to calorie intake versus calories used. Our bodies burn a rate of calories during the day, but if we exceed these calories in our foods without additional physical activity there is a high chance we will gain weight. On the opposite side, if we are in calorie deficit – that is, consuming less calories than our basic calorie burn, plus any active calorie burn – we are likely to lose weight. There are other variables that play a part, including consistency, genetics, metabolism, medical conditions, body chemicals, etc., but essentially, calorie intake to activity is the key reason we lose or gain weight. The main difference is what kind of weight we lose or gain (and where on our bodies), which is particularly important in fitness.

MACRONUTRIENTS

So, as touched on above, quantity of calories needs to be combined with quality and, in particular, the composition of those calories in relation to goals. This is where the old adage "we are what we eat" rings true. The composition of calories, particularly macronutrients (referred to as macros) influences body composition. Macronutrients are proteins, fats and carbohydrates, and they are important in terms of what type of weight we gain or lose.

MACRONUTRIENT

/MAKRƏƱˈNJUːTRɪƏNT/

NOUN

PLURAL NOUN: MACRONUTRIENTS

1. a type of food (e.g. fat, protein, carbohydrate) required in large amounts in the diet.

Alongside your macros are other important nutrients, like vitamins and minerals, plus the need to take in a suitable amount of water.

Protein

Protein consumption is especially important in relation to strength, muscle build, repair, maintenance and reduction. Protein is the body's key building nutrient, not only for muscle, but also for skin, bones, nails, hair, etc. Bodybuilders discovered the importance and benefits of a higher intake of protein for intense training over 70 years ago, even before nutrition experts. Nowadays, it's well-known across all professional sports and recognised and used in everyday (non-pro) fitness training. Protein is formed from 20 amino acids, nine of which are essential (see the amino acids list in the appendix) and obtained through eating certain protein-rich foods, like eggs, milk, and meat. Protein powders, like whey or branched-chain amino acid (BCAA) supplements, which are available in powder and tablets, can also help to provide these amino acids. Experts in bodybuilding go further, saying that to create an optimal anabolic environment for muscle improvement, the correct ratios of these protein building blocks need to be present. However, for the foundations we are building here, let's not get too complicated.

ANABOLIC

Relating to or promoting anabolism.

ANABOLISM

The synthesis of complex molecules in living organisms from simpler ones together with the storage of energy; constructive metabolism.

CATABOLISM

The breakdown of complex molecules in living organisms to form simpler ones, together with the release of energy; destructive metabolism.

A NOTE ON BUILDING VERSUS BREAKDOWN OF MUSCLE:

IN ORDER TO OPTIMISE STRENGTH AND FITNESS, IT'S IM-
PORTANT THAT YOUR BODY IS IN A SUITABLE ANABOLIC (RE-
BUILDING) STATE AS MUCH AS POSSIBLE, OTHERWISE THERE
IS A HIGH CHANCE YOU WILL NEGATIVELY IMPACT PROGRESS.
MUSCLE (AND GENERAL FITNESS) IMPROVEMENT HAPPENS
IN PERIODS OF REST, WHEN THE BODY IS REPAIRING. WHEN
YOUR BODY IS EXERTED THROUGH EXERCISE THE EFFORTS
BREAK DOWN MUSCLE TISSUE, LITERALLY TEARING THE MUS-
CLE, CREATING A CATABOLIC STATE. IF THE BODY DOESN'T
RECEIVE ENOUGH NUTRIENTS FROM CARBS AND, PARTICULAR-
LY, PROTEINS, THE MUSCLE CAN CONTINUE TO BREAK DOWN,
ESSENTIALLY THE BODY "CONSUMES ITSELF". THEREFORE,
IT'S IMPORTANT TO CONSUME ENOUGH PROTEIN, CARBS AND
GOOD FAT TO ENSURE YOUR BODY HAS SUITABLE NUTRITION
FOR EXERCISE, AFTER EXERCISE AND DURING REST, TO HELP
BUILD AND REPAIR MUSCLE. IF NOT, YOU MAY FIND YOURSELF
GETTING WEAKER, NOT IMPROVING.

The important thing is that not all protein sources
are created equal. For example, gram for gram, chicken
breast is a much more amino acid-rich protein source
than soy. Below is a table that shows some common protein sources, the percentage of protein they contain, and
their amino acid score, which is a method of evaluating
the protein quality based on both the amino acid requirements of humans and their ability to digest it.

1. PROTEIN SOURCES & AMINO ACIDS (TOP)
2. PROTEIN SUPPLEMENTS (BOTTOM)

Food	% Of Protein By Weight	Protein Ratings (High = Best Protein Content / Amino Acid Score)
Egg (Whole)	13%	100
Egg White	11%	88
Cow's Milk	4%	60
Fish	18–25%	70
Cheese	22–36%	70
Brown Rice	8%	57
Lean Beef	19–31%	69
Chicken / Turkey	19–31%	79
Soy	42%	47
Whole Grain Wheat	12%	44
Peanuts	26%	43
Dry Black Beans	21%	34
White Potato	2%	34

Supplement	% Of Protein By Weight	Protein Ratings (High = Best Protein Content / Amino Acid Score)
Quality Whey (Isolate)	90%	159*
Quality Whey (Concentrate)	82%	104*
Casein	85%	77

*Bigger Brother is slightly skeptical about these ratings due to the commercial drivers behind the supplementation industry. Generally, consuming high-quality wholefood is likely to be the best option where possible. Supplementation should, as the name suggests, supplement a good wholefood diet.

There are lots of different views and various research studies about how much protein is the right amount. Bodybuilders have long lived by the 2.2g per kilogram or 1g per pound of bodyweight rule, many for over 50 years. However, everyone is different and we all have different objectives. It may take some trial and error to discover what is the right amount for your body without having negative and/or uncomfortable effects (e.g. bloating, irritable bowels and wind). However, if you consume at least 80% of the optimal protein rule (e.g. a 180lb man eating at least 145 grams of protein per day) in most cases you will be OK. If you start to see drops in weight and strength, you may want to up your protein and good calorie intake in increments to see if that helps.

Similarly, while carbohydrates (carbs) and fats are important, it's essential to choose the right ones; for example:

- ☑ Carbs: oatmeal, brown rice, broccoli, sweet potato, banana, blueberries, spinach, etc.

- ☑ Fats: fish oil, almonds, natural peanut butter, olive oil, etc.

Carbohydrates

In the case of carbs, there are simple carbs and complex carbs. Simple carbs (essentially sugars or high-sugar foods) are quickly digested and readily available to the body following consumption. Some complex carbs, like oatmeal, nuts, beans, apples and blueberries, provide slow release energy and contain more soluble fibre, making them better for the body, and they can have benefits such as lowering cholesterol and reducing the chance of heart disease.

However, all carbs are ultimately converted into glucose (blood sugar) with the exception of fibre and glycerine. The most basic carbohydrate our bodies use is a simple sugar glucose, although human bodies also create a more complex carb, glucose, which is stored in muscles and liver as glycogen. In relation to this, some carbs are higher in sugar and digest quicker. This can provide more immediate energy, versus the slower release energy found in a complex carbohydrate, like oats. In training and life, when you consume different types of carbohydrate and for what purpose can be quite important.

Carbohydrates help in the following ways:

☑ Before physical activity: help to increase energy stores and delay fatigue.

☑ During physical activity: maintain blood sugar to fuel the muscles being used.

☑ Post physical activity: replace glycogen and aid recovery.

Simple Carbs

Simple carbohydrates (monosaccharides) are essentially sugars. They are easily digested and can provide a quick boost of glucose into the bloodstream to provide a lift in short-term energy.

Simple carbs can be useful for endurance activity, where the body is in need of fast energy replenishment. For example, a marathon runner or long-distance cyclist.

They are found naturally in many foods:

☑ Glucose and fructose are found in fruits and vegetables.

☑ Galactose and lactose are milk sugars.

☑ Sucrose is common table sugar.

☑ Maltose is a grain sugar.

☑ Examples of simple carbs include; carbonated soft drinks, cakes and baked treats, cookies, cereal, fruit juice, and generally foods containing refined sugar and things like corn syrup.

Complex Carbs

☑ Complex carbohydrates (polysaccharides) contain lots of connected monosaccharides.

☑ Some polysaccharides are digestible, such as glycogen, dextrins and starch.

☑ Other polysaccharides are indigestible. These include cellulose, hemicellulose, pectin, gums and mucilages.

☑ Examples of complex carbohydrates include rolled oats, broccoli, kidney beans, apples, and unrefined grains, like wholewheat bread.

The above is a simple summary of the multi-faceted facts behind carbohydrates, and more detail can be found with a bit of research. However, the key thing for the purposes of this book is, when looking at athletes and fitness training, more conditioned individuals can better convert glucose into glycogen in the muscles. The enzyme in the body that helps to do this is most elevated in the 30-minute window after exercise, so it's important to consume some quality carbs with your protein after a workout to maximise the opportunity.

An additional consideration with carbohydrates is related to the above-mentioned speed at which the sugars enter the bloodstream. This is measured by the glycaemic index (GI) and the glycaemic load (GL) of particular carbohydrates; professional athletes apply a lot of science around this to help sustain energy and improve recovery. Now, measuring the impact of different types of carbs on the bloodstream is a very complex process which we won't tackle here, but the following is a summary which should help to keep you on the right track:

Low-GI foods

☑ These are foods that have a measure of less than 54 on the glycaemic index, which runs from 0 (low) to 100 (high).

☑ These kinds of carbs are absorbed more slowly, have a lower insulin response and are better at helping sustain energy levels for longer periods.

☑ Consuming these carbohydrates can prevent blood sugar from lowering prematurely or too quickly, and reduce fatigue.

☑ Examples of low-GI foods include fruits with fruit sugar (fructose), wholewheat pasta, oats, bran, brown rice and milk (milk sugar – galactose). Most vegetables also have a relatively low GI, except for some, like corn and carrots.

High-GI foods

☑ These are foods that measure 55 or more on the glycaemic index.

☑ These kinds of carbs are absorbed much more quickly into the bloodstream and can create insulin spikes.

☑ High-GI foods can be used to boost energy during extensive training and just after physical exercise, to help benefit recovery, due to their ability to provide a quick energy boost.

- ☑ Consuming higher GI foods within 1.5 to 2 hours of training is known to help replenish glycogen depletion in the muscles.

- ☑ High-GI carbs are often found in highly refined and processed foods, like white table sugar, sweets, white rice, white pasta, white breads and ready meals.

Glycaemic load

THE GLYCAEMIC LOAD (GL) OF FOOD IS A NUMBER THAT ESTIMATES HOW MUCH THE FOOD WILL RAISE A PERSON'S BLOOD GLUCOSE LEVEL AFTER EATING IT. ONE UNIT OF GL APPROXIMATES THE EFFECT OF CONSUMING ONE GRAM OF GLUCOSE. GL ACCOUNTS FOR HOW MUCH CARBOHYDRATE IS IN THE FOOD AND HOW MUCH EACH GRAM OF CARBOHYDRATE IN THE FOOD RAISES BLOOD GLUCOSE LEVELS. GL IS BASED ON THE GI AND IS CALCULATED BY MULTIPLYING THE GRAMS OF AVAILABLE CARBOHYDRATE IN THE FOOD BY THE FOOD'S GI, AND THEN DIVIDING BY 100.

SOURCE: GLYCEMIC RESEARCH INSTITUTE, 2013

NOTE: AS GL IMPACT IS LINKED TO INSULIN AND BLOOD SUGAR CHANGES, THE GI AND GL OF FOODS CAN BE CRUCIAL TO THOSE SUFFERING FROM DIABETES. IF YOU HAVE ANY ISSUES WITH YOUR BLOOD SUGAR, OR EVEN IF YOU'RE UNSURE, IT'S IMPORTANT TO CONSULT A MEDICAL DOCTOR PRIOR TO EXPERIMENTING WITH DIFFERENT FOODS.

As mentioned, this is a complex area, but by looking at the nutrition information of the food and applying some common sense you can quickly start to build an understanding of what foods are more useful for your training and more naturally going to help balance your diet and weight. As a rule of thumb, it's best to avoid heavily refined foods and drinks with lots of sugar and stick to things with less than 10g of sugar per 100g. Also, to get a sugar hit in and around your intense activity, bananas and other natural foods with a higher GI/GL are a better bet. We've included a table with examples of foods and their GI and GL in the appendix and on the Lean Exec website:

BIT.LY/GYINDEX

Fats

In a similar way to carbs and protein, not all fats are created equal. Although in contrast, all fats contain more calories per gram than protein and carbs.

MACRO CALORIES

Macronutrient (MACRO)	Grams	No. Of Calories (kcal)
Protein	1	4
Carbohydrate	1	4
Fat	1	9

Macronutrient (MACRO)	Grams	No. Of Calories (kcal)
Protein	100	400
Carbohydrate	100	400
Fat	100	900

When it comes to fat, don't be a fathead! The reality is that not all fat is bad and, to be really healthy, we need some fat in our diet, even when looking to be lean. Actually, the right kind of fats, assuming sensible consumption, can help you stay lean and some research suggests they can also keep your heart healthy. Fatty acids, like omega-3, are actually crucial to our diet and they help deliver fat-soluble vitamins, provide energy and fuel for the body, plus keep your skin in good condition. The U.S. Department of Agriculture's 2005 Dietary Guidelines stated that we need a minimum of 10% of fat in our daily diet. However, the recommendation is between 20–35%.

The problem is, it's very easy in the Western world to smash through this and hit 40%+ in calorie-dense fats. Not to mention that a lot of the easily available "convenience" foods are full of trans fat, the most evil, artery-clogging of all fats. Eating trans fats (essentially unsaturated fats) regularly and excessively is known to raise your bad (LDL) cholesterol levels and lower your good (HDL) cholesterol levels. Research shows that diets rich in trans fat, increase the risk of Type 2 diabetes, heart disease and stroke.

So, why do fatty foods always seem to taste so good!?! Well, research suggests this can be down to a number of factors, including texture, smell, links to pleasure chemicals produced by the body, genuine nutritional need and cravings. It's also nothing new, so it might be that we are genetically designed to crave calorie-rich food. That seems logical as, if you consider a time when we, as a species, were hunters and gatherers, with food less available, calorie-rich food would be important to survival. In that situation, the appeal of fat makes sense on the basis that fat can be stored as an abundant energy source in the body. In this scenario you can also imagine the benefits of eating nuts, as they are high in calories and fat, gram for gram. Here's a quote which can be found with a search online:

FROM AN EVOLUTIONARY POINT OF VIEW, JUNK FOOD CRAVINGS ARE LINKED TO PREHISTORIC TIMES WHEN THE BRAIN'S OPIOIDS AND DOPAMINE REACTED TO THE BENEFIT OF HIGH-CALORIE FOOD AS A SURVIVAL MECHANISM.

WE ARE PROGRAMMED TO ENJOY EATING FATTY AND SUGARY SUBSTANCES, AND OUR BRAINS TELL US TO SEEK THEM OUT.

TODAY, WE STILL HAVE THE SAME CHEMICAL REACTIONS TO THESE SO-CALLED HYPER-PALATABLE FOODS, CAUSING AN UNIGNORABLE DESIRE – DESPITE THERE BEING LESS OF A NUTRITIONAL NEED FOR THEM.

DR LEIGH GIBSON, READER IN BIOPSYCHOLOGY AT ROEHAMPTON UNIVERSITY

While we have come a long way since then in terms of civilisation, our bodies have not changed as quickly. They still function to optimise our survival. So, while it's become easier to create convenient, delicious foods that have instant appeal with the right kind of marketing, the refinement processes involved to do this and preserve these foods is far from good for us. Not to mention, we eat a lot of it and live much more sedate, stationary lives, particularly those of us who spend a lot of time at a desk. Unfortunately, it's no good blaming civilisation for lack of fitness as, ultimately, we still have a choice. We also have the power to change what we perceive as pleasurable experience and eating.

The reality is it can be a challenge to eat well for training, particularly if you have to change a lot of bad eating habits. However, once you do, the rewards in the way you feel and the progress you achieve will make it worthwhile. In order to get started with your new nutrition regime the first step is to look at your target, set a goal, then understand the macros and calories you need to reach that goal, and what food and supplements you will need to maximise your training plan.

As a starting point, the foods to avoid are vegetable oil, heavily processed meats, supermarket ready meals, sugary cereals, fried chips, white bread and other simple carbs, as well as the most commonly known things, like sweets, chocolate, carbonated drinks, crisps, etc.

On TheLeanExec.com you will find starter plans for eating and also some links to tools that will help you calculate your appropriate macronutrients and calories. These are also readily available online, although it's recommended you use them from a reputable source.

THE RIGHT EATING WITH MINIMAL CHEATING

It's not always easy to manage diet, with a busy schedule and cravings. There are so many factors that can impact an optimal diet schedule. Some include:

- ☑ Delayed commute, stuck in traffic or on a train.

- ☑ Travel for work and travel generally.

- ☑ A meeting that overruns.

- ☑ A new meeting that gets scheduled at a sub-optimal time.

- ☑ A later than usual lie in on a Saturday (following your big squat and deadlift day at the gym, of course).

- ☑ A night out with friends.

- ☑ A romantic dinner with your partner.

- ☑ Your child's activity schedule.

- ☑ A tight deadline.

- ☑ Generally, stuff to do!

The list goes on. Unless you want to give up having a life or staying lean and fit is your job, optimal dieting is difficult. However, these days it is getting easier, as there are more and more foods and supplements on the market (and coming onto the market) that can help reduce the challenge. Even the average supermarket sells ready-made protein drinks and other fitness food products. The Lean Exec methodology, as always, looks to optimise in the best way possible, given the circumstances. We see this in three key areas: food alternatives, meal planning and time-saving solutions (particularly for those times when it's difficult to eat the meals you need and want).

Food Alternatives

The first rule of the training diet is to swap the worst foods you are eating for other delicious foods. It's amazing what an impact this can have (note, the calorie table earlier in the book). For example, eating chip shop fish and chips versus a similar meal bought from the supermarket can make a big difference to calories consumed. Below are some ideas to get you started:

FOOD ALTERNATORS - A

| | Instead of eating... | ...try this... | | ...or better yet. | | Lean Exec | | | |
| | Option 1 | Option 2 | | Home-made Alternative | | Recipe | | | |
	Chip Shop Lrg Fish & Chips	450g Marks & Spencer Fish & Chips	% Diff.	Home-made Fish & Chips w/Panko Breadcrumb	% Diff.	150g Supermarket Cod Fillets, Boneless & Skinless	40g Yutaka Panko Breadcrumbs	100g Aunt Bessie's Homestyle Chips	20g Heinz Tomato Ketchup 50% Less Sugar
Calories (kcal)	1242	750	60%	490	39%	147	150.0	180.0	13
Protein (Grams)	60	31.5	53%	41	69%	32.3	5.3	3.5	0.26
Carbs (Grams)	97	90	93%	67	69%	0.0	35.4	29.0	2.4
Fat (Grams)	68	24	35%	8	11%	2.0	0.8	4.8	0

This home-made option is less than half the calories. The best option is still to eat fish without high calorie batter and/or sauce, but it's a way you can enjoy a favourite without blasting your daily calories off the scale. The downside is this option has less protein, but you can top up 15 – 25g with another low calorie protein source, some peas or even eat another piece of fish within a 750 calorie meal limit. Note – if you are training well and eating well at other meals this is a way you can treat yourself without destroying your goals.

Sources: Sainsbury's | Five Guys | MyFitnessPal.com | FatSecret.co.uk

FOOD ALTERNATORS - B

| | Instead of eating... | ...try this... | | ...or better yet. | | Lean Exec Recipe | | | |
| | Option 1 | Option 2 | | Home-made Alternative | | | | | |
	Standard Byron Burger	Five Guys Burger with ketchup	% Diff.	Lean Home-made Burger	% Diff.	100g Supermarket 5% Lean Mince	Large Egg	Deli Kitchen Plain Flat Bun	20g Heinz Tomato Ketchup 50% Less Sugar
Calories (kcal)	700	520	74%	477	68%	166	78	220	13
Protein (Grams)	35	23	66%	44	124%	31	6	6.3	0.26
Carbs (Grams)	70	44	63%	42	60%	0.5	0.6	38.2	2.4
Fat (Grams)	25	26	104%	14	55%	4.7	5	4	0

The burger has one of the worst reputations in food, but not all burgers are created equal. In fact, in the mix of a good diet, having a standard burger is unlikely to be your biggest problem. However, it will be if you smother it in sauces, like mayonnaise and burger sauce, top it with streaky bacon, cheese and all manner of extras. If you need your burger fix, keep it minimal, particularly at a restaurant. If you do grab a restaurant burger, most will have between 18–30% fat in the meat so pick one with lean meat - it's likely the protein content will also be higher.

Sources: Sainsbury's | Five Guys | MyFitnessPal.com | FatSecret.co.uk

FOOD ALTERNATORS - C

| | Instead of eating... | ...try this... | | ...or better yet. | | Lean Exec | | | |
| | Option 1 | Option 2 | % Diff. | Home-made Alternative | % Diff. | Recipe | | | |
	Dominos Small Classic Crust Pepperoni Pizza	Pizza Express American Pepperoni Pizza (Supermarket)		Home-made Pizza		Sainsbury's Garlic Flatbread, Taste the Diff.	Tomato & Basil Pizza Sauce Topper	8 slices Italian Milano Salami	30g Grated Mozzarella Cheese
Calories (kcal)	1200	704	59%	648	54%	336	51	172	89
Protein (Grams)	52.2	30	57%	31	59%	10.2	1.5	11.6	7.6
Carbs (Grams)	116.4	80	69%	55	48%	46.6	7.2	1	0.5
Fat (Grams)	57.6	30	52%	33	57%	11.4	1.3	13.6	6.3

Sources: Sainsbury's | Five Guys | MyFitnessPal.com | FatSecret.co.uk

The Popular Choice	Lean Exec Options		Notes
	1	2	
White Sugar	Use 20-25% less Demerara or Muscovado Sugar	Honey or Brown Sugar Syrup	Bigger Brother definitely recommends avoiding refined (particularly white) sugar where possible, but we don't necessarily suggest cutting out sugar completely and we'd always recommend small changes first as oppose to sudden dramatic ones. Start by switching to less refined sugar (e.g. Demerara, Turbinado, or Muscovado) and cutting the amount of sugar you use by 20-25%. Interestingly, switching from sugar to honey is often touted as a way to lose weight. In principle this works, but that's essentially because honey only has about 76% sugar vs sugar's 99%. So go figure! Stevia and other low calorie sweeteners are also an option, but why not try these small sweet changes first and see what happens. Note: brown sugar syrup is included here as an option 2, not for nutritional value, but because certain types have 20% less sugar calories per ml/gram than standard sugar.
Full-Fat Milk	Semi-Skimmed Milk	Skimmed Milk	This is an obvious and popular one. Some suggest removing milk from your diet is the best solution. Bigger Brother doesn't agree. Milk is packed with great stuff, not to mention good quality protein, so unless you have a health issue linked to the consumption of milk there is no reason to cut it out of your diet completely. Choose lower calorie milk options and keep consumption through the day moderate and in most cases you'll be fine in the context of a sensible diet. Note: milk (even full-fat milk) is often touted by fitness trainers and experts as a great source of protein and calories for muscle building.

Perhaps more importantly, it's the little changes you make to everyday eating that add up to overall improvements. Try some of these ideas to switch things up:

Butter	Olive Oil based spread	Olive Oil	Unless you are on a mission to have a sub 10% six pack, a small amount of butter in your diet is unlikely to be your nemesis. However, Bigger Brother does recommend avoiding it or keeping it to tiny amounts daily, e.g. a very small amount spread thinly on your toast.
Mayo	Under 15g of light Mayo	Don't use it if you are using Butter or Cheese	Similar to butter, if you are training well or unless you want to be a fitness model, a bit of mayo (e.g. 15-20g a day) here and there won't destroy your progress.
White Bread	Brown, Rye and Oat options	Bagels	Gluten and carbs generally have a bad reputation these days. There is no shortage of diets telling you to cut your bread and carbs. Obviously, if you have a health aversion to these things, you may need to avoid them in what you eat. However, if you are training regularly, some bread and carbs are not going to be your biggest problem. In fact, they can help give you the energy you need to train well and burn off some extra calories. Like with everything, if you keep it in moderation in an overall diet and choose healthier options, bread can still be enjoyed.
Replace your average Cereal...	with good quality Porridge Oats	or Shredded Wheat	Not only will oats make you feel more full, they are super-healthy and give you loads of great energy. You can even add some demerara sugar or honey, just try to keep it under 7-8 grams a serving.
Porridge with Milk	Porridge Cooked in Skimmed Milk	Porridge Cooked in Water	All we get is gruel! A neat trick to reduce calories and still have a tasty porridge is to cook the porridge in water, then add a little cold skimmed milk and a few grams of demerara sugar. This tastes fine and the reduced milk content will mean less calories.

FOOD ALTERNATORS - TREATS
And how about some tricks for these treats?

The Popular Choice	Lean Exec Options 1	2	Notes
Milk Chocolate & Chocolate Bars	Go dark and choose a less sugary option	Keep it to 2–4 squares, no more than once or twice a week	The reality is, chocolate is often packed full of fat and sugar calories, but it's not all bad. Research has shown that chocolate can lower cholesterol levels, improve insulin sensitivity, is good for the brain and makes you feel better. Choose dark chocolate with higher amounts of cacao and less sugar.
Beer	Less Beer	Occasional Beer	Bigger Brother likes beer and drinks it regularly! However, if it's not enjoyed in moderation it will limit progress. Beer and alcohol is generally full of empty (non-nutritious) calories. If you drink it daily and to excess regularly it will inhibit your progress. Keep it in check and it will not only improve your Lean Exec progress, but also your overall efficiency and productivity in daily life. Don't refrain from enjoying yourself, just try to keep drinking to once or twice a week. Eat really well the day before/day after, drink water in between and, if possible, get some good rest after drinking and before heading to the gym for a good session the next day. Unofficially, if you are generally getting the right mix of macro calories in your diet, a few beers may even help you get the extra calories needed for pushing up size and strength. However, this is not an excuse to drink more!

Ordering Takeaway	Don't eat Takeaways	Don't eat Takeaways	Come on people! Really!? Not only are takeaways an expensive way to eat, most are packed with gut-wrenching poor choice calories. Many of your favourite dishes will smash through your daily calorie count in one fell swoop. If you must eat convenience meals, keep it to occasional treat days or find an oven-heated supermarket alternative. Better yet, save your calorie blaster meals for date night at a favourite restaurant and get the squats in the next day to leverage all those calories.
Your favourite Restaurant Dishes	Keep it to occasional Treats and enjoy it when you do eat it	Go with less Sauce, leaner cuts of Meat (e.g. Rump Steak), drop the Starter, Dessert or both	Bigger Brother loves eating out and doesn't always hold back, life's too short! Just try to keep it to occasional treats, then you can enjoy it without guilt. If you know you're going out for dinner that day, make sure the rest of your day's eating is clean and lean. Also, why not do a big training session the next day to leverage all those calories?

Tips & Tricks

☑ Possibly an obvious one, but go for the leanest meats (and get your quality fat requirements from other good sources (e.g. eggs or avocados):

- Go for chicken breast, as opposed to leg or thigh meat. It's packed with protein and low in fat (as long as it's not smothered in a fatty, sugary sauce) and usually a top option. If you want to go even leaner, turkey is also not just for Christmas. Turkey has even less fat than chicken and is available as breast and mince in many supermarkets. Bigger Brother especially likes turkey bacon. Tasty and lean.

- Avoid pork and lamb, which typically have higher fat content. Exceptions can be bacon medallions and lean ham cuts. Good lean meats have 20-25+ grams (30+ grams in the best) of protein and under 5 grams of fat per 100 grams, although note that the salt content can be high. If you like lamb, save it for treat meals.

- Choose your minced beef wisely. Most supermarkets now offer mince with varying levels of fat. While it's better to eat red meat less often than, say, chicken and fish, a lean 5% mince is not a bad option.

- Steak! Bigger Brother loves a good steak. Sadly, some of the most delicious cuts, like ribeye, are high in artery clogging fat. Go for lean cuts, like rump (20g+ protein per 100g) or, if you've got the budget, fillet (25g+ protein per 100g). Cuts like this also have typically less than 15g of fat per 100g.

NOTE: FOR MEN OVER 25 AND PARTICULARLY OVER 40 (WHEN TESTOSTERONE LEVELS START TO DIP), RED MEAT CAN HELP BOOST TESTOSTERONE LEVELS NATURALLY – SO IT CAN BE BENEFICIAL TO HAVE IT IN MODERATION.

☑ If you're making something like a sandwich that could taste better with butter, cheese and mayonnaise, then as well as keeping it minimal and choosing low calorie ingredient options, you can cut out just one or two of these. Often, you only need one of these ingredients to give your food pep and losing the other two keeps the calories lower.

☑ Cheese is often demonised. However, there are a lot of different varieties of cheese and lots of leaner versions of traditional favourites available. It's generally better to keep cheese consumption to a minimum (i.e. to maybe three times a week) and if you need a fix, go for cheeses like feta and buffalo mozzarella. There are also some great lower-fat options that are a bit like classic Emmental.

It's also best to avoid heavily processed cheeses, e.g. sliced cheese (like the ones used in McDonald's and Burger King burgers), Dairylea, Cheese Whiz, etc.

☑ Adding something high fat to your meal? Drop the carbs, and vice versa.

☑ Use small (10ml max) portions of olive oil for cooking, instead of other cooking oils. If you want to minimise calories, switch to an olive oil or avocado cooking spray.

Meal Planning Starters

You can find some ready-made meal plans and helpful meal planning calculators, tools and other useful resources on The Lean Exec website:

BIT.LY/EATNOCHEAT

Time (& Money) Savers

☑ Home-made protein milk. Make some powdered skimmed milk mixture and add 10–20g of unflavoured high-quality whey protein powder. Mix it up with a powerful blender and let it settle. Add some frozen blueberries, known for their superfood antioxidants, or a banana.

☑ Cook extra food at dinner time and take the leftovers for lunch, e.g. roast a chicken and spread it across 2–4 meals.

☑ Cook up some lean burgers with 5% fat mince, 2% fat chicken or turkey mince. If you measure them out to 100–150g each, it's an easy way to be sure you are getting a good 30–40g of protein.

☑ Go hunting in the frozen section of the supermarket for kale, spinach and ready-made veggie smoothie mixes. Add some water and maybe a bit of fresh apple juice, blast it in the blender. Make enough so you can keep it in the fridge or freezer and have a shot once or twice a day over three days. Just ensure it's not too sugary. This is a great way to get some high-quality nutrients quickly and without many calories.

☑ Frozen veg is known to have similar nutrient values as fresh veg. Keep it in the freezer and microwave for a quick, low calorie, nutrient-dense complement to your nicely spiced chicken breast.

☑ Invest in some compartmented Tupperware. As you're cleaning up after dinner, get your leftovers straight into the plastic containers, put in the fridge and it's ready to grab and go in the morning.

☑ It's all gravy, baby! Instant chicken and even beef gravy is a great way to get some flavour without too many calories. All it takes is a teaspoon or two and some boiled water. Drizzle over your chicken to taste.

THE CORE EXERCISES

As you probably guessed, this section is all about the core exercises that you'll need for The Lean Exec (Symmitarian) training. As mentioned, the approach is designed to minimise complication, reduce excess gym time and get the most bang for your workout buck. Therefore, it's not an endless list of isolation movements and fancy fad exercises. These next few pages detail the exercises and structures we know, over many years of training, deliver the best balance of effort in, to results out. There may be a point in the future where you want to add some variation (although that doesn't mean a dramatic shift from the core approach), so we've also added a link to an alternative moves table for when you feel like a change or the equipment isn't available. See the Alternative Moves table on the website: BIT.LY/ALTMOVES for options on each exercise.

CORE CARDIO EXERCISE
Jog/Run

It's most likely that you have a concept of jogging/running and have exercised in this way before in some form (if not as an adult, at least in the playground or PE at school). Therefore, we'll focus on key techniques and form that will make your running more efficient, effective and lower your risk of any injury.

NOTE, RUNNING IS A BIT OF A CATCH-22 WHEN IT COMES TO IMPACT. EXERCISES LIKE RUNNING WITH MORE IMPACT CAN CAUSE JOINT AND MUSCLE PAINS AND STRAINS, OR WORSE FOR SOME PEOPLE. HOWEVER, IMPACT CAN BE A GOOD THING AS IT HELPS MAINTAIN BONE MASS WHICH IS REALLY IMPORTANT IF YOU WANT TO COMBAT THE EFFECTS OF BONE DENSITY REDUCTION DUE TO AGING. SADLY, BONE MASS PEAKS AROUND 30 YEARS OLD AND DECLINES FROM THERE AS OUR BODIES AGE.

WHILE ALTERNATIVES TO RUNNING LIKE SWIMMING AND CYCLING CAUSE LESS IMPACT AND ARE HELPFUL FOR FITNESS, THEY DON'T "CHALLENGE" THE BODY THROUGH IMPACT IN THE SAME WAY, SO WON'T NECESSARILY HELP IN THE MAINTENANCE OF BONE DENSITY AS WE AGE. FIRST AND FOREMOST, YOU SHOULD SEEK YOUR DOCTOR'S ADVICE IF YOU ARE UNSURE IF RUNNING IS SAFE FOR YOU. IF IT IS, BUT YOU ARE STILL CONCERNED ABOUT THE IMPACT, FOCUS ON BUILDING AT YOUR

PACE. THIS DOESN'T MEAN YOU SHOULDN'T PUSH YOURSELF, JUST BE MINDFUL TO DO THIS GRADUALLY, FITNESS IS A JOURNEY, IT DOESN'T HAVE TO BE A RACE. YOU CAN ALSO DO THINGS TO MINIMISE ANY RISKS, LIKE ENSURING YOU HAVE THE RIGHT RUNNING SHOES FOR YOUR FEET, GETTING QUALITY SPORTS INSOLES FOR YOUR SHOES, STRETCHING, ENSURING YOU ARE ALLOWING APPROPRIATE TIME FOR RECOVERY, ETC.

☑ Foot landing: it may seem trivial, but the particular way your foot hits the ground while running is very important. The aim for landing is to ensure your toes are pointing down, with your foot at a natural angle so the ball of your foot can land first, followed by a roll backward to the back heel. You really want to avoid a flat-footed landing, where your foot is parallel to the ground. It's also good to focus on a speed and rhythm that allows you to use this technique to minimise direct impact with the ground. The light landing and roll to the heel should cushion the landing and you should not let the whole of your heel touch the ground. Focus on creating a smooth and natural "cycle" with your feet landing, rolling and lifting in a smooth revolution. If you have used an elliptical/cross trainer machine before, try to imagine recreating the low impact movement of its cycle with your feet as you run.

☑ Lower body (legs, back and hips, particularly): the power of your run comes from your quadriceps and, more broadly, your legs and hips. These are the muscles that will help propel you forward. It's important to keep the body stable and controlled without any unnecessary side-to-side movement. Stay relaxed and keep your posture generally straight/upright, only succumbing to the slight natural lean forward that the movement creates. Don't go too far forward as this bend at the waist can increase the potential for lower back impact and pain.

☑ Upper body: while the lower body does most of the work during a run, the upper body is also important for good form. Keep your head and neck in a natural upright position, looking forward (don't look down at the ground in front of you). Your back should be relaxed, with your arms bent and elbows at your sides. Your hands should be in front of your body. Keep your hands comfortable, slightly closed, palms facing in position or in a relaxed fist. Keep your arms within this basic position, only moving them back and forth gently with the rhythm of your run. It's important to keep your arms light and relaxed but controlled. Minimising the movement to just enough to meet your run rhythm will give you a fluid motion, but also use your body's energy more efficiently, with the main resources being used to focus on the run.

☑ Breathing: the aim with breathing while running is to try to have a steady, deep rhythm. Breathe deeply and naturally through the mouth, lifting and releasing, while allowing your diaphragm to fill with air. Doing this also helps to contract your abs and can work your midsection, in tandem. If you're struggling with breathing, try to use your running steps to create a pattern for inhaling and exhaling in a comfortable way.

Notes

☑ If you'd rather not run, cycling, playing a sport that involves cardio (e.g. football/basketball), or using a stationary bike or elliptical/cross trainer will also work. Just note the points about impact. If your goal is to increase your strength and/or muscle size and you're not seeing strength improvements during the conditioning stage and you're doing more than 1.5 hours of cardio per week, try cutting down your cardio and/or checking your calorie intake is enough for your exercise regime

☑ Alternatively, or in tandem, it may be the case that you need to up your intake of good calories to compensate for your additional exercise. Or get more rest. More on this later in the book.

Interval Training (Altenative to Jog/Run)

If you are feeling confident and want to up the intensity of your cardio with maximum effect, you can try interval training. Running intervals are a common training method for 100 metre sprint athletes, and have you ever seen a pro sprinter that doesn't have a lean muscular body? The great thing about interval training is that it's great at burning fat and maintaining muscle, as opposed to longer distance running that not only loses fat, but generally loses weight all round (including muscle mass) by cannibalising the body for energy. There is lots of science to show this, but you only have to look at the difference between pro athletes who run 5,000 metres+ and athletes in the sprint range of 100–200 metres, and even 400 metres, to see this in effect. Essentially, sprinting is about raw power for short bursts; whereas it's not advantageous for the body to carry any mass, even muscle mass, for long distances.

So, what exactly is it and how do you do it? A simple approach to interval training is essentially jogging at low intensity for 60–120 seconds, then sprinting at full capacity for 20-30 seconds. You repeat this cycle of jog then sprint for 10 minutes or more depending on your fitness. You can do this while road running or cycling, but it can be easier to control using a treadmill, stationary bike or elliptical trainer.

For more on cardio and exercise options, go to: BIT.LY/TLE-CARDIO

CORE BODY WEIGHT EXERCISES

Body Weight Squats

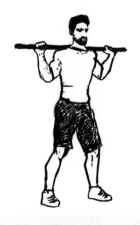 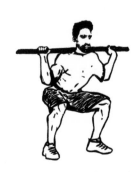

1. Starting position: stand with feet a comfortable shoulder width apart.

   A. You can place your hands behind your head (elbows out), or;

   B. Hold your hands out straight in front of you, or;

   C. Use a lightweight bar (or even a broom handle) across the shoulders (see diagram).

2. Keep your body posture straight. Look forward, keeping your head straight, breathe in, then bend your knees (as if sitting) until your bum is in line with or just below your knees.

3. Push from your heels and straighten your legs, returning to the starting position, breathing out to complete the squat.

4. Repeat.

Notes

☑ Bodyweight squats are sometimes referred to as Air Squats.

☑ Be sure to keep your back in a natural arch and your chin up, facing forward throughout the movement.

☑ If at first you struggle to go low enough to complete the squat, go as low as you can, while still being able to return to the starting position without losing form. However, always do your best to try and complete the move. It's not meant to be easy, so try to grit your teeth and push to the max your fitness will allow. Fitness is about mental strength, not just physical.

☑ Depending on your fitness and flexibility, this may be hard at first. However, if you follow this guide, each time you do an exercise session try to push yourself further than the previous session. The first time it may be just pushing yourself to complete one whole rep with good form, but soon you will have to use increased repetitions to challenge yourself.

☑ If you cross your arms in front of you and perform body weight squats it can also be an effective warm up and dynamic stretch.

Standard Push-Up

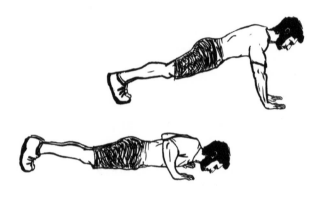

1. Kneel down on the floor and place your hands in a comfortable position, just wider than your shoulders.

2. Starting position: extend your legs and rise up onto your toes. Ensure your body is straight, like a plank angled down from your shoulders to the floor, where your toes are bent to support your lower body.

3. Breathe in as you bend your arms and lower your chest to the floor.

4. Push your body up using your arms and return to the starting position, breathing out as you complete.

5. Repeat.

Notes

☑ Be sure to keep your back straight and hold your body firm during the movement.

☑ If you struggle to go low enough to complete the push-up, go as low as you can, while still being able to return to the starting position without losing form. However, always do your best to try and complete the move. It's not meant to be easy, so try to grit your teeth and push to the max your fitness will allow. Fitness is about mental strength, not just physical.

☑ Depending on your fitness and flexibility, this may be hard at first. However, if you follow this guide, each time you do an exercise session try to push yourself further than the previous session. The first time it may be just pushing yourself to complete one whole rep with good form, but soon you will have to use increased repetitions to challenge yourself.

☑ If you are really struggling with a full push-up, then try doing a partial push-up, with knees resting on the floor, or even a movement similar to the Upward Dog (see below) until your arms are strong enough to complete a push-up.

☑ You can also try lying on the floor and pushing yourself up as far as you can, resting, then trying again, for the appropriate number of sets and reps. If you do things like this enough you will eventually get strong enough to do full push-ups.

Pull-Up

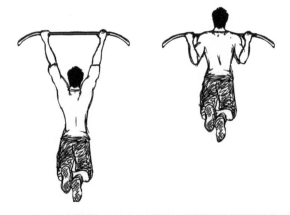

1. Reach up and grab the pull-up bar, with your hands in a comfortable, natural position, about shoulder width apart or slightly wider. You can face your palms towards you or away from you, but it's recommended to use palms facing forward at this stage in the training.

2. Starting position: hang from the bar with arms extended. You can leave your legs dangling together in a natural position or, alternatively, cross your legs at your ankles and bend your knees to pull your legs up. If the bar is quite low for you, then bending your knees and crossing your legs may be necessary to complete the move without touching the floor.

3. Looking up, draw the shoulders and the upper arms down and back, pulling your chest up towards the bar until the bar touches your upper chest (or as close as you can). Your neck and head should be over the bar height.

4. Hold for a second, then lower your body down to the starting position, with control, to complete a repetition.

Notes

☑   Be sure to keep your body as steady as naturally possible and try to complete the move with control.

☑   If at first you can't complete a full repetition, there are two things you can do to work yourself up to complete the move:

   ▪ Grab the bar, as highlighted above, and use your legs to jump and push yourself up until your chest is at the bar (as described in points 3 and 4). Try to lower yourself as slowly as possible, with control, as described in point 4 (a negative rep). If the bar is too high to easily jump up to, use a stable box, crate, step or supportive object to assist.

   ▪ You can use an assisted pull-up machine in a gym, reducing the supportive weight in each session until you can complete a rep without assistance. Unless you are really struggling to gain progress each session, we would recommend trying to use the negative rep option as it can be more effective at improving strength and pushing past boundaries faster.

☑   The negative rep method can also be used to push a final rep, once you cannot complete any more full repetitions with good form. This can help push your progress for the next session.

☑   Depending on your fitness and flexibility, this may be hard at first. However, if you follow this guide, each time you do an exercise session try to push yourself further than the previous session. The first time it may be just pushing yourself to complete one whole rep with good form, but soon you will have to use increased repetitions to challenge yourself.

Parallel Bar Dips

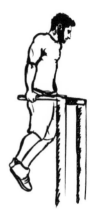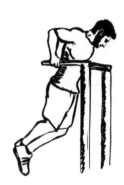

The (tricep) dip is a great compound movement and a Bigger Brother favourite. Not only can they really work your triceps, but they also hit your chest and shoulders!

1. Starting position. Grip the bars with your hands and push yourself up (you can use a little jump if it helps) until you are holding your body straight up above the bars. Your arms should be locked straight at your sides, supporting your weight. Keep your feet together and bend your knees slightly to keep your feet from touching the floor, if necessary.

2. Inhale as you bend your arms and lower your body until your elbows reach a 90-degree angle. Keep your elbows close to your body and your torso as straight as possible to focus on the triceps. Now, inhale and slowly lower yourself downward.

3. Exhale and use your arms, focusing on your triceps, to push yourself back up into the starting position. You have completed one rep.

Notes

☑ If you've completed the conditioning phase of this training plan you should find it easier to complete at least one rep. However, as with any body weight exercise, the first time you try can be difficult; stick with it and you'll soon see your reps increase. If you're really struggling, you can use the weighted dip machine to assist until you have developed more strength.

☑ You can cross your legs at the ankles, but be careful that this doesn't force you to lean further forward. A forward lean will hit your chest more, but within this plan you need to concentrate on hitting your triceps.

☑ More advanced lifters will sometimes add weight, using a weight belt, to really hit their triceps hard.

Ab Crunch

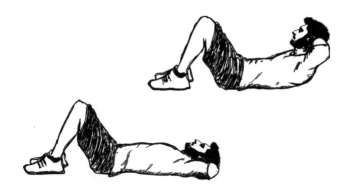

1. Lie with your back flat on a mat or directly on the floor. Keep your feet about shoulder width apart and bring your knees up, so the bottoms of your feet/trainers are flat on the floor. This should be a relatively comfortable position.

2. Lightly touch your temples with your fingers, with palms out. Your elbows should be pointing out to the sides, away from your body. This is your starting position.

3. As you exhale, bring your shoulders and upper back off the ground until you feel a tense in your abdominal area (this is the crunch!).

4. Hold for a second or so, as you tense the abs, then in a controlled manner, lower your upper back and shoulders back down to the starting position.

5. Repeat this for the desired number of repetitions.

Notes

☑   This is the classic ab move and should be all you need until you are more advanced, particularly if you are doing your core training correctly.

☑   The ab muscles get worked in many exercises, so if you can't see a decent set of abs and it's important to you, it's more likely that you need to increase cardio, reduce calories, or both, rather than do more ab exercises. You can have the greatest abs in the world, but if you can't see them for fat, it's no use!

☑   The Lean Exec training doesn't involve much direct ab work as it's all about optimal bang for your buck or, in other words, results for time. If you are doing your other training correctly, your abs will only need a bit of additional polish and crunches will do the job until you are more advanced.

☑   If you really want to do more abs, as they are small muscles you can work them almost every day, or at least every other day. Just make sure you listen to your body and, if it doesn't feel right, take a breather.

Plank

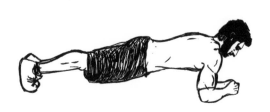

Unless you're walking off one of them on a pirate ship, planks aren't that exciting. However, the plank is great for your core strength, shoulders, arms, glutes and, generally, your posture.

1. As if you are going to do a push-up, get down on your knees and place your hands on the floor, in a comfortable position, just below your shoulders.

2. Extend your legs and rise up onto your toes. Then, bend your arms and get down on your elbows, with your hands in fists, almost touching each other at the knuckles, below your head (crone re a triangle with your upper arms).

3. Ensure your body is straight, like a plank angled down from your shoulders to the floor, where your toes are bent to support your lower body.

4. Hold for as long as you can. You should be targeting a minimum of two minutes.

Upward Dog

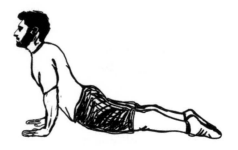

While you may not want to do yoga, this is one of many moves from yoga worth exploring. It's great for stretching your back and ensuring you're flexible and avoid injury doing those squats and deadlifts.

1. Get down onto the floor (use a mat if preferred) as if you're about to do a push-up, but rest your thighs/legs on the floor and point your toes out (top of foot resting on the floor). Use your bent arms, with your hands placed under your shoulders to support your upper body/torso. This is the starting position.

2. Using your arms, push your upper body up until your arms are comfortably straight (slight bend at the elbow). Keep your thighs and legs on the floor as you do this, and

stretch, with the natural curvature of your back. You can face forward or look up.

3. Hold this position for 20–45 seconds (or as long as it feels comfortable). Then return to the starting position.

4. Repeat this three times, or until you feel your lower back is comfortably stretched.

Child (Restful) Pose

Another one from the world of yoga, this is a great way to stretch the hips, thighs and lower back, helping to keep you limber for those squats and deadlifts. In yoga, it's also seen as a great way to reduce stress, relieve back/neck pain and restore balance to the body. Executed correctly and regularly, it will help relax muscles while gently stretching the back and upper body (torso).

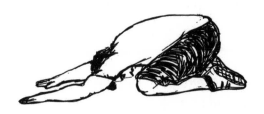

1. Kneel on the floor.

2. Spread your knees comfortably wide and point your toes away from your body. They should be close together with the end of your toes/shoes touching or almost touching.

3. Lower your glutes onto your heels, then sit up straight, keeping the natural curvature of your back.

4. As you exhale, bow forward, stretching your arms out in front of you, as if you are praying to the gym god!

5. Hold this position, with your arms extended with a gentle stretch, and palms facing down.

6. Gently press back with your hands to keep your glutes in contact with your heels.

7. Feel the stretch across your back, stretching it wide and relaxing your lower back.

8. Hold the pose for as long as you feel comfortable. Then, when you are ready to release the pose, gently use your hands to guide you back to sitting on your heels.

Notes

☑ **Try experimenting with different hold times and repeat the pose a few times each session, if you wish.**

WARNING: AVOID DOING THIS POSE IF YOU HAVE A KNEE IN-JURY OR THERE IS ANY RISK OF INJURY OR EXACERBATING AN ISSUE. THIS SHOULD BE A CALM, RELAXING STRETCH, SO IF YOU HAVE PAIN IT'S ADVISABLE TO CONSULT A DOCTOR.

SIU PRINCIPLE

Now that we've summarised the core body exercises, it would make sense to introduce the SIU Principle – **Suck It Up Principle!!**

I often hear people moaning (even personal trainers) that they can't do a pull-up, push-up, plank or whatever, and the answer is to look for an alternative move. Now, unless you have some kind of injury, health issue or other legitimate excuse (note: not being strong enough is not an excuse), then there is no excuse. The best way to overcome the inability to do these great exercises is to *try* doing it until you *can* do it! If you're learning to ride a bike, do you stop when you can't do it and just give up? No, you keep trying until you can do it! The same thing applies to most new things in life.

When I did my development day for my fitness instruction and personal trainer course, I had to do a pistol squat in front of 12 people. If you don't know what a pistol squat is, have a look at videos online, but it's essentially a one-legged squat, with your other leg pointed straight out in front and your arms straight out in front for balance.

It was the first time I'd ever tried it and, despite doing barbell back squats with 100kg+ for multiple reps every week, it was extremely difficult to do it effectively. I was impressing no one with this gun, but I had to Suck

It Up! The point is, no matter how trained you get, when you try something new it is nearly always tricky at first. However, it's surprising how effective the body is at learning and, if you are persistent, you will soon get it and often the first period after that is the best time for rapid improvement.

So, when you first start something new, don't expect to necessarily enjoy it, and don't just give up and try something easier – you generally need to remember the Suck It Up Principle and keep trying until you can do it. That's life!

CORE RESISTANCE TRAINING EXERCISES

Deadlift

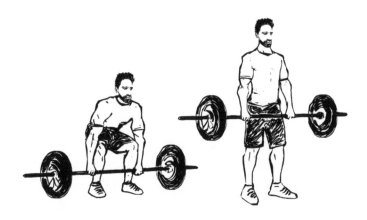

A strong body starts with a strong core. There are lots of discussions as to which weighted exercise is the ultimate move, and Bigger Brother believes, from experience, that the deadlift is the move that can make any man or woman solid as a rock. Although squats are awesome too, mastering the deadlift is perhaps trickier and can really help advance wider success in the gym. That's because it not only requires very important focus on form, but also hits the body like no other move can. The deadlift not only hits the legs (quads and hamstrings), glutes and lower back (erector spinae and quadratus lumborum), but also the forearms, middle back, lats and traps. Bigger Brother has also found it hits and strengthens hands, arms and wrists (at least, when pushing up the weight level), as, effectively, you are still holding up a heavy weight with arm tension, even if they don't move much. So, if you think you have weedy wrists or forearms stop training them and start deadlifting. Your wrists and forearms won't be weak for long! Ultimately, this is a great move to help you build overall body strength and muscle. If you don't believe it, just go online and search Hugh Jackman, Henry Cavill, Arnold Schwarzenegger, Ronnie Coleman or Franco Columbu "Deadlift", and have a look at the images!

Now, while it's important, it can also be challenging and even daunting, so it's absolutely crucial to learn the correct technique to avoid injury. Once you have the correct technique, it allows you to push your lifting, and it's shifting that heavy weight that will get maximum results. Therefore, it makes sense to practise the correct technique with a very light weight (e.g. bar only, or even a broomstick handle) and then try increasing until you are confident that you have the technique right and can perform the lift correctly with a very challenging weight.

It's also important to note that this move also hits the nervous system and lower back hard, so it may only be necessary to do this move once per week with heavy weight, at least until you are very experienced. By the way, by "experienced", this means lifting 180-200% of your body weight, depending on your height and weight. In addition, if you're tall (over 6ft) this can be even more challenging as you have longer limbs and have to move the weight further. If nothing else, learn to listen to your body. Soreness and some discomfort can mean progress, but if something feels painful or "wrong", exercise caution.

Correct Technique

1. Load up the barbell with a weight that you're confident you can lift.

2. Starting point: approach the bar and stand in front of the bar with your feet about hip width (no more than shoulder width) apart. Your lower legs should be close enough that you are almost touching the bar with your shins. Keep your back as straight as possible, head up, looking forward. Bend at the hip and grab the bar with both hands about shoulder width apart (on the outside of your knees). Your legs should be bent comfortably so you can reach the bar and shoulders should be protracted (forward) naturally.

NOTE: IF YOU ARE LIFTING A WEIGHT THAT IS PARTICULARLY HEAVY FOR YOU, TRY REVERSING ONE HAND SO YOUR PALM IS FACING OUTWARDS. THIS ALTERNATE PALM TECHNIQUE GIVES YOU BETTER GRIP FOR LIFTING HEAVIER WEIGHTS. BIGGER BROTHER SUGGESTS ONLY DOING THIS WHEN YOU CAN'T LIFT

THE WEIGHT WITH A PALMS INWARD GRIP. IF YOU ARE NEW TO DEADLIFTING, WE RECOMMEND STARTING WITH LOWER WEIGHTS AND USING A PALMS INWARD GRIP UNTIL YOU ARE COMFORTABLE YOU CAN LIFT SOLIDLY WITH GOOD FORM.

*Very important: before you lift, make sure your neck and head are up and you are looking straight ahead. While doing this, also ensure your back is straight, shoulders up, with the natural curve in your lower back. If your back is rounded and hunched, this is very bad form and can put you at high risk of injuring your back. If you have a chest logo on your T-shirt you should be able to see it when looking in the mirror.

3. With your feet and grip in position, breathe in and lower your hips into a semi-squat where your butt (gluteus maximus!) is just above your knees (don't go to a right angle or low like a full squat). As you flex your knees, your shins should touch the bar and you should feel some tension in the back of your legs. With your chest and head up, look directly ahead and keep the natural curve of your back. Now start lifting, pushing from the ground, where your feet and heels are firmly planted. As you move from bent knee position, engage your upper body and arms, ensuring you maintain a straight back, head-up form until you reach a standing, upright posture as you breathe out. Stand to attention, like a soldier, with your arms straight down in front, holding the bar. Ensure your shoulders are straight back in a natural good-posture position, not

hunched forward. While you should have a slight lean back at the top of the move, don't lean too far back. The body should be straight, taut, shoulders back (slight squeeze between the shoulder blades) and thighs pressed against the bar. Stand to attention!

4. Return to the starting position by bending the knees and moving the torso forward, maintaining the straight back form used for the first part of the lift. Once the weight is back on the floor, you have completed one rep.

Notes

☑ This is not a move to do lightly. If you have back issues, it would be best to consult your doctor beforehand. While the author cannot offer, and this does not constitute or substitute, medical advice, he found starting with a low to moderate weight and building up the weight each week actually helped to resolve some persistent lower back pain. In the case of the author, by focusing on the deadlift once per week he was able to go from having regular back pain and lifting less than 50kg to lifting well over 100kg in less than 12 weeks (in test, I can now do 20 reps with 100kg). Note, the lower back problem was resolved within the first month or two.

☑   In any case, with this lift, be absolutely certain you have the form correct before lifting weight. Also, get to know yourself and your limits cautiously. This doesn't mean you shouldn't challenge yourself (in fact, you should), but ensure that you don't do anything that will break your form, as it could cause serious injury if executed incorrectly. If in doubt, use a lighter weight than you think you can lift and use a one rep max calculator to monitor your max ability.

☑   Some people also use straps and there are techniques used by powerlifters to enhance ability to lift heavier weight. However, unless you are aiming to be a powerlifter and compete, Bigger Brother doesn't recommend this. Our philosophy is to use your body and use the best possible form, versus using additional aids. If you prefer to wear gloves, go for it, although thin rugby type gloves with no padding are best. Try to keep it as raw as possible, at least in the early days. It's not essential, but flat shoes (e.g. Converse canvas shoes or powerlifter shoes) or even bare feet can be good for deadlifting.

☑   If you are finding this move particularly hard and daunting, you can try using dumbbells or a trap bar to build up your confidence.

☑   As this move can hit the nervous system hard, it can be beneficial to take a week off deadlifting every 4–6 weeks. This recuperation period can also be useful in breaking plateaus and pushing your deadlift onwards and upwards. The main thing is to learn to listen to your body. Challenging yourself is important, but an injury can be a major setback to hard work.

Squat (Barbell)

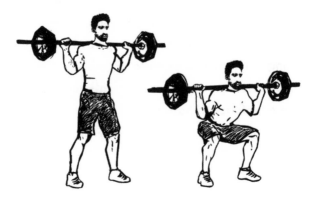

As you've probably figured out by now, Bigger Brother loves the deadlift and unofficially crowns it king of the gym moves. However, we also love the squat! The main reason we see the squat as second-in-line to the throne is because while it hits the legs, gluteus maximus and lower back significantly, it doesn't hit areas like the forearms, middle back, lats and traps. If you're just starting with deadlifts and squats and only feel comfortable doing one, Bigger Brother always recommends building up your deadlift first, particularly as, once you add in squats, you will not only find that you have a reasonable starting squat due to the deadlifting, but also the new impact the squat adds to your workout will give you some shock leg improvement that will even push up your deadlift.

As with the deadlift, though, squats with weights shouldn't be taken too lightly (pardon the pun). In some ways, squats can be riskier than deadlifts. For example, while attempting a heavy deadlift, letting go of the barbell may create a huge noise as it hits the floor, but having your legs collapse under a squat or dropping a heavy weight off your back has an increased chance of causing a severe injury. While it's not essential to have a spotter for squats, you might find it useful at the beginning. More importantly, Bigger Brother definitely recommends using the safety bars on a squat rack to ensure that in the unlikely event something does happen, you're not going to have a heavy barbell come crashing down on you. Just make sure the safety bars are low enough for you to complete a full range of motion.

Generally speaking, and as mentioned for the deadlift, it's important to be cautious with the weight until you have a grasp on the level of weight you can manage. The good thing is that even using lighter weights the first few times you squat (or do any new exercise, for that matter) can reap rewards as the introduction of the different weighted movement tends to impact the body anyway. If you want to test a new weight level you could try limiting your range of movement (only going as far down as you dare, to see how it feels). Despite what hardcore squatters say about the importance of going low, you can still get benefit from semi-squat movements, although don't make it a habit, concentrate on good form with a lower, manageable weight and build up over time.

Correct Technique

1. As mentioned above, it's recommended that you perform a barbell squat using a squat rack and apply the safety bars.

2. Set the bar in the rack around shoulder height. Choose a rung on the rack that is low enough that you can easily lift it off the rack rung and high enough that you only need to bend slightly to get your shoulders under the bar.

3. Step under the bar and place your shoulders (slightly down from the neck) at the centre of the bar. Grip the bar with both hands, about halfway between your shoulders and the sides of the rack where the bar is resting. This should be a comfortable, natural arm position with your arms out to the side.

4. Ensuring that your head is up and your back is straight, with a natural curvature of the spine, lift the barbell from the rack by pushing your legs and then your torso, while straightening your body (your legs may be slightly bent). Once the barbell is released from the rack rung where it was resting, move backwards slowly by stepping backwards.

5. Starting position: your legs should be around shoulder width apart and your toes should point slightly outwards. Your body should be supporting the full weight of the bar without any contact with the rack. Very important: *ensure your head is up/looking forward and your back is straight at all times.*

6. Inhale while you slowly lower the bar by bending your knees and hips, while maintaining a straight natural posture with your back. Keep your head up and look forward, while you drop your butt down to the knees or ideally just lower than your knees. Your calves and upper legs should be at slightly less than a 90-degree angle – this is the bottom of the squat. To avoid putting unnecessary pressure on your knees and to hold good form, the front of the knees should make an imaginary straight line with the toes, not go past the toes.

7. From the bottom position, exhale and drive up with your heels and legs until you are standing in the starting position. You have then completed one rep.

Notes

☑   As with the deadlift, be sure to always perform this move with good, accurate form to avoid injury. Get used to the movement with a lighter weight and get to know your strength before attempting it with challenging weight levels.

☑   Everyone has a different body, so don't force an extremely low squat because it looks like the experienced squatters are doing it. Find your "low point" and try to improve it with lighter, manageable weights.

☑   If you currently have back issues or have suffered from back issues in the past, it's advisable to consult your doctor before performing this exercise. While this exercise can help strengthen your back significantly and help avoid further back issues, it's important to use extreme caution until you know your back is strong enough to support and lift a particular weight.

☑   While there are other variations of the squat with different foot positions, Bigger Brother recommends sticking with the standard squat until you have a reasonable level of experience.

☑   If you have completed the conditioning phase body weight squats, as recommended, and you start with a very low to moderate weight on the barbell, you should be fine. However, if you are finding the barbell squat daunting, you may want to try doing weighted squats with kettle bells (or dumbbells) either held at your sides or one held with two hands on your chest, to build up confidence and practise getting the squat technique correct with weight.

☑   As mentioned above, some hardcore squatters would say you should only do squats with full range of motion. While this is generally true and it's good to practise full range of motion on most sets, if you have reached a plateau or want to try to push your squat weight up, Bigger Brother has found that trying a heavier weight and only doing a partial rep with limited range of motion (as low as you dare) on your first two sets, then completing your further sets with a lower weight and full range of motion can help bring on the hypertrophy. It can also help put that little extra pressure on the quads, if it's an area you want to strengthen. However, this is not an excuse to be lazy and you should not make this your regular approach.

Leg Curls

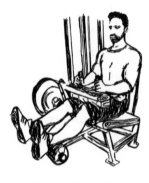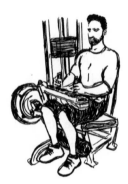

1. Adjust the seat back rest to suit your height, then adjust the leg curl rollers so the back of your ankles (just under your calves) can rest on the pads when you sit on the machine. Adjust the thigh pad down enough that it's touching the top of your thighs when seated, but is not restrictive. Set the desired weight.

2. Sit on the machine with your back against the pad, your legs stretched out with a slight bend, the backs of your ankles (just below the calves) resting on the leg curl roller pads and your hands on the handles of the thigh pad (you can put your palms on the top of the pad, if preferred). Adjust the thigh pad further, if necessary. This is your starting position.

3. Exhale as you use your legs (flexing your knees) to pull the machine lever down and as far back as you can towards your thighs (in a quarter circle motion). Keep your upper body in a stationary position, with your back against the seat pad. Hold the weight for a second or so.

4. In a controlled manner, return the lever and weight back to the starting position, breathing in through this part of the movement.

5. Complete the repetitions.

Notes

☑ This can feel like an awkward movement. Start with light, easy weights and after a few sessions it will start to feel a bit more comfortable. Alternatively, try the lying leg curl machine.

☑ Warning: it's generally best to work with lower, manageable weight, as forcing a larger weight with this exercise can easily shift into poor form, putting unnecessary pressure on sensitive areas like the lower back.

☑ Bigger Brother prefers to use this or lying leg curls as a support exercise, alongside core, multi-joint movements, like back squat and deadlift. If you've already worked hard on squats and deadlifts, a few sets of leg curls will really ensure you've hit your upper legs all round.

☑ If you are feeling solid and want to push your progression, you can try doing 4–5 sets of leg curls before your squats and deadlifts, to ensure you are really giving your hamstrings a workout during those core movements. However, approach with caution! If you tire your hamstrings, squat with extra care and ensure you can manage the weight.

Calf Raises

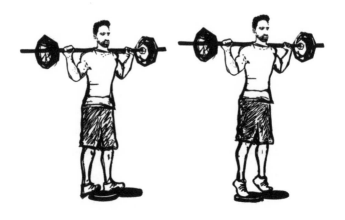

Calf raises are one of the few isolation moves that Bigger Brother recommends from the start. Most people neglect training their calves and find they need to play catch up with the rest of their body later-on. If you naturally have small calves (like me), there is a high chance that calves will be one of the hardest muscles to increase in size, mainly because, like the legs in general, they are used to hard graft, carrying your body all over town. In the beginning, and when you are pushing hard, you may find that your calves are getting a nice workout just from the deadlift and squats, but by including some calf raises you will ensure these muscles grow strong and keep up.

What apparatus you use might come down to what is available in your gym. If you have one, Bigger Brother recommends the standing calf raise, where you stand with your toes on the ledge and the top of your shoulders against the pads and push up with the ball of your foot. However, use the best calf raise you have available. You may also find it works to use a Smith machine bar on your shoulders and a step to recreate the calf raise machine, or do your calf raises on a leg press.

One thing that can be really important is to use the right amount of weight. You may find quite quickly that you are doing calf raises with a significant amount of weight, but not getting much hypertrophy or growth. As mentioned above, by nature, our legs are used to more punishment than our arms, as they are carrying us around all day. If you reach the max weight on the calf machine and can lift multiple times, try shifting to an alternative calf exercise or drop the weight a bit and increase the reps. You may find higher rep ranges of 15 – 20 work better for calves and legs generally.

Correct Technique

1. Adjust the apparatus to fit your height or, if seated, your leg length.

2. Starting position: if you are using a standing calf raise, put your shoulders underneath the pads. If seated, sit back in a comfortable position, in line with the seat. Place the balls of your feet on the ledge or foot pads provided and ensure

your knees are slightly bent. Your toes should face forward in the standard position and your heels should be down in relation to your toes. As you get confident with this move, you can try different foot positions, such as toes facing in or out.

3. Push off the balls of your feet and raise your heels as you breathe out. You should feel a tension in your calf muscles. Hold briefly and then breathe in as you return to the starting position with a controlled drop of your heels. You have completed a rep.

Notes

☑ If using the standing calf raise or doing this move standing, ensure you keep your posture straight to avoid unwanted injury to your lower back. If you have lower back trouble, you may find it best to use a seated calf raise option until your back is fully recovered.

☑ As mentioned, there are a number of different variations of the calf raise and at least one is usually available in most gyms. It's important to follow the instructions shown on the relevant fitness apparatus in your gym.

☑ Ensure you allow the heels to go low and feel a stretch in the calves at the top and bottom of the movement.

Bench Press (Plus Variations)

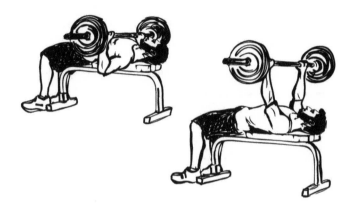

The bench press is perhaps one of the most famous muscle training moves, second only to the bicep curl. As a tool for building a Superman physique, the bench press is in many ways a superior exercise. As a compound movement, it's a key factor in developing a strong upper body. Mastering the bench press using free weights, whether that be barbell or dumbbells can really pound out results. If it was only possible to do three weighted movements to develop a physique, the bench press would be up there with the deadlift and pull-downs for all round power, mass and symmetry.

Correct Technique

1. Adjust the bench to a flat or inclined position. Place the barbell on the rung of a bench press rack at a level where you will be able to lift it off the rack.

2. Lie back against the bench, under the barbell placing your feet flat on the floor in a comfortable position either side of the bottom of the bench. Your back should be straight on the bench, with the natural arch of the spine. It's helpful to lightly push your upper back and shoulders into the bench. The barbell should be above your eye level while in the rack, so that when you take it out of the rack it's directly above the middle of your chest. Grip the barbell with both hands, about medium width, either side of the bar (between your headline and where the barbell is resting on the rack).

3. Starting position: lift the bar off the rack and hold it above your chest with locked, straight arms supporting the barbell weight.

4. Breathe in and lower the weight, with control, until the centre of the barbell brushes your chest. If you are doing a flat bench press then this should be across the centre/ middle of your chest (pectoral) area, with your arms at 90 degrees to the side.

5. Hold for a second, then breathe out as you push the bar back up to the starting position. Ensure that as you push the focus is on squeezing (contracting) your chest

muscles. Maintain this contraction as you straighten and lock out your arms. After a second, lower the weight again to your chest. You could technically count the repetitions from the starting position or the chest position. Bigger Brother tends to count from the chest position.

6. After completing your reps, return to the straight arm starting position and place the barbell back into the rack.

Notes

☑   Take longer to lower the weight (around twice as long) than to press the weight.

☑   This move is not to be taken lightly. The last thing you want is a heavy bar dropping on your chest. It's advisable to train with a spotter, but in all cases using the safety bars in the rack equipment is recommended. If you don't have a spotter or safety bars, it's probably best not to go too heavy with the weight or, alternatively, to use dumbbells, so you can easily drop them at the side.

☑   Don't bounce the weight off your chest. It should only lightly touch your chest at the bottom of the move.

☑   There are different variations of the bench press, but until you have a reasonable level of mass and strength, Bigger Brother recommends you stick to medium grip and only alter the incline.

☑ Some people would argue that it's better to train with a barbell than dumbbells. Bigger Brother would say it's good to train with a barbell in a bench press rack, but using dumbbells can be just as effective, particularly if you train alone and want to push the weight without worrying about possibly being pinned by a bar. Whatever your combined dumbbell press, most likely you will be able to press a similar or even slightly higher amount with a barbell.

☑ You may sometimes see experienced and unexperienced lifters drop their elbows lower than 90 degrees when doing a dumbbell/bench press. Most likely the unexperienced lifter doesn't realise they are engaging their upper back in the movement. Experienced lifters may be doing it to maximise the stretch on the pectorals. The only way you can know for sure is if you ask them.

Lat Pull-Down

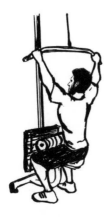 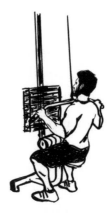

The lat pull-down machine is one of the few machines in the gym that makes you wish it could be classed with "free weight" status. While, in most cases, working with free weights over machines is superior, the lat pull-down is a glorious exception. If you want strength, size and a back that matches your chest, the lat pull-down is a great best friend. Not to mention that the lat pull-down can be a useful tool in building great biceps and shoulders.

Correct Technique

1. Sit down on the lat pull-down machine seat and adjust the knee pad so the front of your upper legs (quads just above the knee) are snuggled comfortably under the knee pads. This is to help keep your body in a seated position while you perform the exercise.

2. Reach up and grip the bar with both hands, using a medium arm width (around the point where the bar curves down). You may need to rise up slightly off the seat to do this and your palms should be facing forward. Ensure you're seated – the weight of your body should be enough for you to sit with arms extended, holding the weight. This is your starting position.

3. Using your arms and focusing on squeezing the back muscles, breathe out and bring the bar down to your chest by pulling your shoulders and arms down and back. If you are performing a standard lat pull-down, angle your torso back about 30 degrees, stick your chest out (peacock style!) and ensure a natural and safe curvature in your lower back.

4. Hold for a second, while you squeeze the shoulder blades together (to stretch your back and lats) then inhale as you slowly (about twice as slowly) use the opposite motion to return the bar back to the starting position. You have completed a rep.

Notes

☑ There are different variations you can do with grip width, palm position and angle. The straighter you are, the more work your biceps will do. Each variation can be used to focus on different objectives, but Bigger Brother recommends sticking to a medium to wide (just past shoulder width) grip with the angles shown at this point in your training.

☑ Bigger Brother doesn't recommend the behind-the-neck version unless you are an experienced lifter as this can put unnecessary pressure on the rotator cuff and isn't essential to developing your back and arms

☑ The straighter your body position, the more you will work your biceps and the less you will work your back.

☑ Minimise the use of forearms, they should just act as levers. Although when you are lifting heavy you will notice the forearms taking the strain, particularly in the final reps.

☑ Grip styles can vary from use of the thumb, as in gripping a bike handle, to using the fingers as a "hook". You can use the style you want at this stage, but Bigger Brother recommends the hook version, leaving the thumb out of it (or loose), as this helps to minimise use of the forearms.

Seated (Cable) Rows

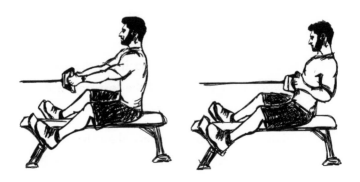

Seated rows are great for building strong arms and a solid back. If you're looking to thicken out your upper body and beef up your arms, heavy rows can really do the trick. If you're not looking to gain thickness, drop the weight and increase the reps to get a solid workout which will make you strong to the core. Bigger Brother also likes machine rows (particularly wide grip), although we tend to do these towards the end of a session, after completing core exercises.

Correct Technique

1. You can do this move with a variety of grips, but to get started, grab the V-bar. The V-bar (palms facing each other) is relatively neutral and should be a comfortable position

tho grip for most people. Attach the V-bar to the low pulley on the cable row machine. To get started, put both feet comfortably on the foot plates (or bar) and keep your knees bent slightly.

2. While maintaining the natural alignment (curve) of your back, lean forward with a gentle stretch to grab the V-bar handles.

3. Keep your arms extended, holding the V-bar, and pull back to a seated position (torso at 90 degrees to your legs).

NOTE: USE CAUTION, PARTICULARLY WHEN THE WEIGHT IS HEAVY, AND ALWAYS ENSURE YOUR BACK IS MAINTAINING ITS NATURAL CURVE, NOT HUNCHED OR STRAINED UNNATURALLY. YOUR BACK SHOULD BE SLIGHTLY ARCHED WITH YOUR CHEST STICKING OUT (YOUR BEST JOHNNY BRAVO IMPRESSION). YOUR LATS SHOULD FEEL TAUT. THIS IS YOUR STARTING PO-SITION.

4. To begin the repetition, breathe in, then pull the V-bar back towards your torso, keeping your upper body stationary. You should pull the bar back until your wrists essentially touch the abdominals and your lower ribcage. Breathe out as you do this.

5. Ensure you squeeze your back muscles and feel the tension. Hold the contraction position for a second, then return to the starting position (point 3) in a controlled manner – i.e. you should be using a weight that is difficult, but not beyond your control.

6. Once you return to the starting position, you have completed one repetition. Continue to complete the repetitions required for the set.

Notes

☑ Avoid swinging your upper body back and forth as you can cause a lower back injury if you're not careful. It's very important to exercise caution with your back on this exercise and ensure you maintain a straight, natural lower back curve at-all-times.

☑ If you aren't totally comfortable with performing a seated cable row (or you want some variety), you can also try machine rows, to build confidence. Just make sure that you set the machine so it allows you to do a maximum range of motion to get a full stretch.

Seated Machine Rows

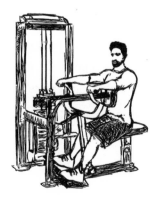 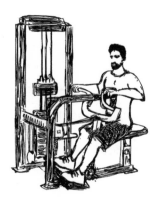

Bigger Brother also likes seated machine rows. These are a nice alternative to cable rows. They are slightly more isolated, due to the reduced flexibility of the machine, but can be a great addition to a workout. These machines often have a palms facing (hammer), medium and wide grip options. Bigger Brother likes to go wide and really stretch the muscles.

Correct Technique

1. Fix the torso/chest pad to a position that is comfortable, but when your feet are on the footrests it's a stretch to reach the grips.

2. Sit on the machine, put your feet on the footrests. While maintaining the natural curvature of your back, lean

forward and grab the grip handles. Take the strain of
the weight with your arms. This is the starting position.
Breathe in.

3. Breathe out as you pull back in a controlled manner until
your hands are parallel to your chest. Stick your chest out
against the torso/chest plate. Hold the contraction, stretch
the chest, squeeze between your shoulder blades and lats.

4. Return to the starting position. You have completed a rep.
Now continue the reps until you finish your set.

Notes

☑   This is one of the few machines that Bigger Brother
really likes to complement free weights. It's great
for control and stretching the muscles. This is a
move that we like to increase the reps on and
often use it as a session-finisher.

☑   This is a great opposing move to the bench press
or seated chest press.

Seated Shoulder Press (Dumbbells)

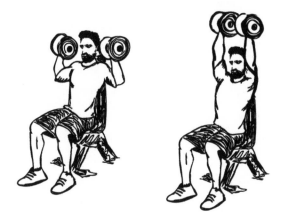

The shoulder press, whether performed with dumbbells or a barbell (military press), is a real Bigger Brother favourite. It's a great compound movement that will help you develop strong shoulders. In addition, as part of a workout with lat pull-downs and bench press, you're hitting the shoulders (and even triceps) from all angles. As you may already have realised, great shoulders make for a muscular and larger looking physique.

1. Pick up your dumbbells (ensuring you keep your back straight and that you don't hunch your shoulders). Sit down on a bench with an upright back support. Keep your back straight, with the natural curvature of your lower back. You can rest the dumbbells on your knees (upright), particularly if they are very heavy for you, or pull them up to an upright position under your chin, palms facing in, using your forearms to support them.

2. If you can, use your strength to push the weights up (with some momentum) so they are either side of and just above your shoulders (palms facing forward, elbows out). If this is difficult, you can rest them on your thighs and use your thighs to push and propel the dumbbells up, with momentum, one at a time. You're now in the starting position.

3. Exhale, pushing the dumbbells up above your head, and touch them lightly together above your head. Hold for a second and contract your shoulders, then slowly lower your arms, bringing the weights back to the starting position, inhaling on the way down. You have completed one rep.

Notes

☑   There are a couple of different ways to do a shoulder press, including standing military press with a barbell and Arnold's variation, the Arnold Press, where you start with your palms facing in (supinated) and rotate out as you move into the traditional press. You can also do a shoulder press, like the above, but standing up, although for people with lower back problems, less experience or an undeveloped back, using the bench as support is recommended.

☑   It's very important to exercise caution with your back on this exercise and ensure you have a straight, natural lower back curve against the bridge..

Side Lateral Raises

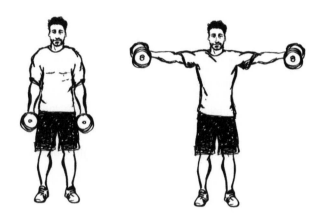

This is another one of the few isolation moves Bigger Brother recommends getting into early in your training. The compound movements in the plan hit your shoulders from all angles quite effectively while you're building up some strength and mass. However, this is a nice move to ensure your shoulders are going to grow nicely all round! In addition, building up the outer part of the shoulder is going to give you that extra bit of width that will add to an Apollonian physique (wide shoulders to slim waist) that is often seen as more aesthetic (the classic example is one of the pioneers of modern bodybuilding and one of the people that inspired Arnold, Steve Reeves).

Correct Technique

1. Grab a pair of dumbbells, being careful to keep your back straight. Stand upright, with good posture (ideally in front of a mirror so you can watch your form) dumbbells in hand either side (palms facing inward) by your outer thighs. This is your starting position.

2. Using controlled movement and focusing on your outer shoulders, keep your torso stationary and exhale as you raise your arms up in an arc, elbows slightly bent and with your hands tilted slightly forward. Raise your arms until they are shoulder height and parallel to the floor.

3. Inhale as you lower the dumbbells back down to the starting position. You have completed one rep.

Notes

☑   It's recommended that you execute this movement in a standing position, but you can also do it seated on a bench. Just be sure to keep your back straight and sit upright, with good posture.

☑   If you reach a plateau with lateral raises it can be worth trying cheat reps with a particularly heavy weight for one or two early sets. This involves using dumbbells that you will only be able to lift halfway through the full range of motion. You should only do one or two sets with low reps and complete the rest of your sets and reps using a strict movement and full range of motion, with a challenging weight.

Barbell Curls

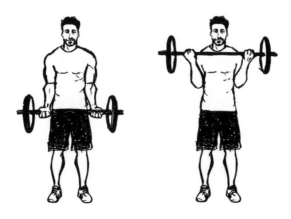

If biceps were a celebrity, they'd likely be the kind that gets lots of column inches and PR, without having the most talent. Essentially, biceps are often seen as the prime sign of manly strength. However, in reality, they are quite small muscles in relation to other muscles, like the chest or even triceps. Often, when people (particularly guys) go to the gym for the first time, they start doing dumbbell curls. It looks cool and due to "bicep fame" it's assumed that if you build bigger biceps you will have big arms. The reality is the triceps (a three-headed muscle, versus the biceps, which is a two-headed muscle) play a much bigger part in arm size.

That's not to say you should ignore biceps, but when you're looking to build up your bicep mass, rather than doing lots of dumbbell curls in different variations, getting good at doing barbell (or EZ-bar) curls with heavy weight and good form is going to get you better growth results. Not to mention that, until you are more developed (and by more developed, I mean a good 190lbs+ of lean muscular mass!), compound movements like pull-ups and lat pull-downs are going to do a lot more for you than isolation movements. Plus, it helps to avoid many of the mistakes people make with symmetry. You want the body to look as proportional as possible within your genetics. Getting big biceps is great, but not if you look strange because they are too big for your back, chest and triceps!

If you have limited options in your gym or training environment, curling two dumbbells or using an EZ curl bar will also work, but Bigger Brother recommends getting good at barbell curls with different grip widths.

Correct Technique

1. Load the short Olympic barbell 152cm (5ft)) and weight 16kg (35lbs) – not the deadlift bar!) or EZ-Bar 8-11kg (25lbs) on the floor with your chosen weight.

2. Approach the bar, bend your knees, keep your back straight (a deadlift posture is good for this) and grab the bar with your palms facing outward a comfortable shoulder width apart.

3. Stand up, keeping your back straight and using your deadlift technique to avoid injury. This should be easy as you will be used to lifting heavier weight with a deadlift.

4. Starting position: stand upright, with good posture. You should be holding the bar with straight arms (a comfortable

shoulder width apart), palms facing out, with the bar level to your upper thighs.

5. Breathe out as you keep your body straight and curl the bar up, focusing on your biceps. Your elbows should stay at your side and only your forearms should move, in an arc, upwards. Continue all the way up until the bar is level with your shoulders. Squeeze your biceps at the top.

6. Inhale as you slowly lower the bar back to the starting position. You have completed a rep.

BIGGER BROTHER ALSO LIKES REVERSE GRIP (PALMS FACING DOWN) BARBELL CURLS AS THESE CAN REALLY HELP FOCUS ON THE BICEP LENGTH AND ALSO HIT THE FOREARMS HARDER, TO DEVELOP OVERALL ARM STRENGTH. FOR A VARIATION, ALSO TRY WIDER GRIPS TO HIT FROM A DIFFERENT ANGLE.

Notes

☑ As mentioned above, you can do this movement with dumbbells or an EZ-bar, although straight bar is the classic bicep building mass movement.

☑ If you have no other options, you could use a straight bar attached to a low pulley machine or bicep curl machine, but if these are your only options you might want to find a new gym!! Remember, an expensive gym with fancy equipment won't necessarily make you strong and muscular. Most impressive and powerful bodies have been built with hard work and basic free weights.

Tricep Push-Downs

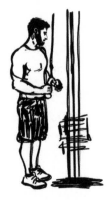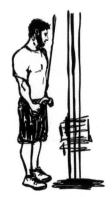

After tricep dips, and other compound movements (in the plan) that hit the biceps, this is an isolation move worth getting into early on. Learning how to do this properly will give you that extra hit that means your biceps will develop at pace with the rest of your body.

Correct Technique

1. Using the pulley machine, attach a straight or (upside down) V-bar to the high pulley.

2. Starting position: grab the bar with both hands, about shoulder width apart, palms facing down, and lean forward slightly, with one foot a little in front of the other. Your elbows should be pointing down and the underside of your forearms towards the pulley machine, in front of you.

3. Keeping your body steady and your elbows tight against your ribcage, exhale, as you push the bar down until your arms are fully extended towards the floor and the bar is touching your thighs. Focus on equally contracting the triceps during the movement. Only your forearms should move.

4. Hold for a second and, as you breathe in, return to the starting position, using the opposite movement. You have completed a rep.

Notes

☑ There are a couple of variations using the straight-bar, EZ-bar and rope attachments, amongst others. Bigger Brother recommends using the V-bar where possible, especially if you notice wrist pain/strain using a straight-bar.

☑ It's recommended that you switch front foot forward on each set and be sure that you are focusing on the triceps area equally for both arms in this exercise.

☑ If you don't have access to a pulley machine you can substitute this exercise with standing dumbbell or EZ-bar triceps extensions.

Standing Overhead Triceps Extensions (Bar or EZ-Bar) – AKA The French Press

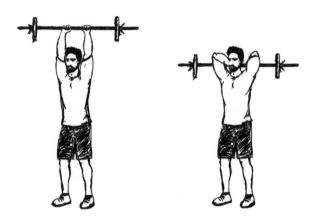

This is a great triceps move that also hits the shoulders and your arms generally. As you're standing (ensure your back is in a natural curve) supporting the weight, it will indirectly improve your core.

1. To start, get into a position similar to a deadlift (hands should be knuckles out, palms in). Maintaining the natural curvature of your back, feet about shoulder width apart, pick up the bar with your hands a comfortable hip width apart and get into a standing position. The bar should be resting at the top of your thighs, with your arms straight, but not tensed, comfortably holding the bar.

2. Hoist the barbell or EZ-bar above your head, holding the bar straight up with a natural, fully extended, but comfortable position, elbows slightly bent. This is the starting position for the rep.

3. Ensure your upper arms are close to your head, not touching, but parallel to your ears. Lower your forearms using the natural motion of your elbow until the bar is behind your neck. Your biceps and forearms should be touching. Keep your upper arms (biceps and triceps) flexible, but stationary, elbows pointing slightly out. Don't forget to breathe in as you lower the bar.

4. Feel the muscles tense and stretch, then push the bar back (with the natural motion of the elbows) up to the starting position, maintaining the upper arm position. Breathe out as you push the bar up.

5. That's one rep; now repeat until you have completed the number of reps for the set.

Notes

☑ You can also do this move holding one side of a dumbbell (facing down), a triceps bar (palms facing each other) and appropriate cable machines, using a bar or rope.

☑ As with most moves in the gym, take care not to put the wrong kind of strain on your back. A standing move will help build your core, but you should always ensure you can manage the weight and maintain the natural curvature of your back.

☑ For variation, you can also try performing this move seated on a bench.

Machine (Butterfly)
Fly & Reverse Machine Fly

This is a great Symmitarian machine to really wrap up a workout. Although the front machine fly is essentially a chest machine, Bigger Brother likes to sit low and use it after core shoulder moves, leveraging front and back in succession to really stretch the chest and hit the shoulders all round.

Front Fly

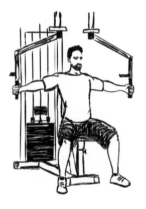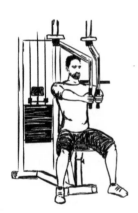

1. Adjust the arms of the machine so they are on the furthest front setting or, if you can manage it and it's comfortable, go one notch further for a really good stretch.

2. Adjust the seat so it's low enough that your arms can go straight out to the sides, near parallel to the floor.

3. Sit on the seated area with your back against the pad, maintaining the natural curvature of your back.

4. Grip the handles. Your arms should be stretched out (your best Jesus pose) and possibly slightly back, if you have gone for the widest setting. This is your starting position.

5. Keeping your arms relatively (comfortably) straight, push the handles as if you are creating a semicircle in front of you. Breathe out as you perform this part of the movement, squeeze the chest and hold the contraction for a second or so.

6. In a controlled manner, return to the starting position, ensuring you get a wide chest stretch.

7. Repeat this until you have completed the desired number of reps.

Reverse Fly

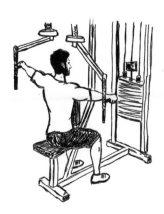

1. Adjust the arms of the machine so they are on the furthest-back setting and select a suitable weight.

2. Adjust the seat low enough that your arms can go straight out (shoulder height) in front and to the sides, near parallel to the floor.

3. Grip the handles, palms facing in towards each other. Your arms should be straight out, directly in front of you. This is your starting position.

4. As if at the centre of a semicircle, pull the hands out to the sides, keeping your arms comfortably straight (arms slightly bent at the elbow) in a semi-circular motion until your arms are stretched out to your sides parallel to the floor. Breathe out during this part of the movement. Stretch and squeeze the upper centre of your back, contracting your rear delts.

5. Hold this for a second or so and then, in a controlled manner, return to the starting position.

6. Repeat for the appropriate number of reps.

Notes

☑   It's not essential that you grip the handles on the front fly. A loose grip is fine, but you can also keep your palms/hands flat and push the handles with the centre of your palms.

☑   You may find you are naturally stronger one way or the other. Bigger Brother suggests using the max weight of your weaker side to try to maintain a balance.

☑ Generally, we do these in succession, e.g. front, then back, then rest.

☑ In our training approach, we tend to use the machine fly as a finishing move, using a lower weight and working in higher rep ranges of 12–20.

Alternative Moves

As mentioned, The Lean Exec approach is aimed at simplifying, rather than complicating. It's designed to minimise time and maximise results. Generally, it makes sense to stick to the core exercises, but sometimes equipment isn't available and/or you just need a change. You can access an alternative moves table on The Lean Exec website, which will help you vary exercises without deviating from the Symmitarian Way.

View the Alternative Moves table on The Lean Exec website:

BIT.LY/ALTMOVES

In addition, the website also includes some alternative training plans based on the Symmitarian principles. You can view them here:

BIT.LY/TLE-PLANS

ONE REP MAX

If you didn't know already, your one rep max (1RM) is your one repetition maximum. In weight training/lifting, it's the maximum amount of force that can be generated in one maximum contraction or, in other words, the heaviest weight you can lift once, correctly and completely.

For example, if you can bench press 100kg once, for one full repetition, and it's not possible to do another full repetition, then your one rep max or 1RM is essentially 100kg. This can be a useful stat to track your progress and it's often referenced in The Lean Exec training, although it's not necessary to actually do it (unless you want to). In fact, arguably testing your 1RM can be dangerous, if you don't do it correctly or safely. For example, if you overestimate your strength and try to lift a very heavy weight off the bench free weight rack, then can't support it or find the strength to put it back on the rack, you could drop the heavy weight on your chest, causing serious damage.

We don't want to deter you from trying it at all, just ensure you do it safely, using a capable training instructor or partner (spotter) who can help you if you get into trouble, or by applying the safety bars that are now available with most modern equipment. Ideally, you should do both, but if nothing else, it's recommended you use the safety bars.

If you don't fancy testing your 1RM just yet, or would rather not do it for any reason, there are other ways to check this stat with a lighter, more manageable weight. A quick search online will show there are lots of calculators available that will allow you to input a weight you can lift, say, 5 or 10 times, that will then give you a reasonably accurate estimate of your 1RM. There are also lots of gym mobile apps that allow you to input your lifting progress and estimate your 1RM and other useful stats, like volume of weight lifted automatically.

Here are some suggestions on the website to get you started:

BIT.LY/TLE-1RM

LEAN EXEC TRAINING PLANS

These workouts should be followed as described, although it's really important to try to listen to your body. If it feels wrong it often is, so just exercise caution and take your time, it's a journey not a race. You should also try experimenting with a week away from the gym every month or two using the hours for other activities. These could include bodyweight plans like the groundwork training or other sports like football, swimming, rollerblading, surfing and skiing, or whatever interests you as long as it's physically active. This should be active rest from the gym, not an excuse to watch more Netflix!

Let's get started...

GROUNDWORK PLAN (WAX ON, WAX OFF)

In this conditioning period of 4–12 weeks (depending on your starting fitness state and progress) there are four key exercises to complete in each training session, 3–4 times per week.

Work Out: 4–12 Weeks' Conditioning

COMPLETE 3–4 TIMES PER WEEK, WITH 1 DAY'S REST BE-
TWEEN EACH SESSION. EACH SESSION SHOULD TAKE AROUND
50 MINUTES AND NO MORE THAN 1 HOUR.

Basic Warm-Up | Stretch

- ☑ **Quad Stretch:** Hold for 10–15 seconds and repeat for both legs

- ☑ **Lunge:** Hold for 10–15 seconds and repeat for both legs

- ☑ **Lateral Lunge:** Hold for 10–15 seconds and repeat for both legs

- ☑ **Shoulder Stretch (Across Chest):** Hold for 10–15 seconds and repeat for both arms

- ☑ **Tricep Stretch:** Hold for 10–15 seconds and repeat for both arms

- ☑ **Upward Dog:** Hold for 10–15 seconds, repeat 3 times

- ☑ **Child Restful Pose:** Hold for 10–15 seconds, repeat 3 times

NOTE: AS MENTIONED IN THE SECTION ABOUT WARMING UP,
STRETCHING AND COOLING DOWN, YOU MAY FIND DYNAMIC
STRETCHING USEFUL. MORE ON THE WEBSITE, HERE:
BIT.LY/TLE-STRETCH

EXERCISE PLAN

MOVE	SET	REPS	% OF 1REP MAX	LOW TARGET REPS	HIGH TARGET REPS	GUIDE TEMPO	REST PERIOD AFTER SET (SEC)
1. Standard Body Squats	1	To Failure	Body Weight	10	20	2010	60
	2	To Failure	Body Weight	10	20	2010	60
	3	To Failure	Body Weight	10	20	2010	60
	4	To Failure	Body Weight	10	20	2010	75
	5	To Failure	Body Weight	10	20	2010	75
	6	To Failure	Body Weight	10	n/a	2010	75
Total				60	100		
2. Standard Push-Up	1	To Failure	Body Weight	8	15	1111	60
	2	To Failure	Body Weight	6	15	1111	60
	3	To Failure	Body Weight	5	10	1111	60
	4	To Failure	Body Weight	4	10	1111	90
	5	To Failure	Body Weight	4	10	1111	90
	6	To Failure	Body Weight	3	n/a	1111	90
Total				30	60		
3. Standard Pull-Up	1	To Failure	Body Weight	6	12	1020	60
	2	To Failure	Body Weight	5	10	1020	60
	3	To Failure	Body Weight	4	8	1020	60
	4	To Failure	Body Weight	3	6	1020	90
	5	To Failure	Body Weight	2	5	1020	90
	6	To Failure	Body Weight	1	4	1020	90
Total				21	45		

Jog/Run

Finish your workout with a 20-30 minute run at a reasonable pace, in line with your fitness. You should be sweating and tired at the end of the run, but it's important to run at a pace that will allow you to complete the whole 20-30 minutes.

NOTE: IF YOU FEEL CONFIDENT, THE INTERVAL TRAINING IS SUGGESTED AS AN ALTERNATIVE TO THE JOG/RUN.

If you really don't like running, replace with other cardio exercises - e.g. Cycling, X Trainer, Stair Climbing, Rowing or anything you enjoy.

A NOTE ABOUT THE GYM TRAINING PLANS

The 3-Hour Power Plan is refined based on the routines I did to lose 10kg of fat and change my body composition over eight weeks to a leaner more muscular first phase of The Lean Exec. The additional plans are refined based on the ongoing training after this initial stage.

I've aimed to make it as simple and concise as possible, based on what I know can work with the right effort and commitment. However, depending on your body, eating habits, fitness, strength, sleep quality and schedule, you may need to take the insights from earlier in this book and modify the exercises and routines to best suit your personal situation.

As I can't be there in person to review your status and help you tweak things, it will be down to you. But that's OK; just take your time, start at a level you can manage and then increase as and when it doesn't feel like it's enough. Keep pushing yourself a bit harder each week. The key is to use the plan as a guide and discover what works for you. Don't cheat yourself by not pushing yourself enough (remember, intensity is important) equally if you overdo it you may risk injury. You need to find the balance at your personal edge and learn when to keep going and when you're done on a particular day.

Here is an example of how you can adjust the 3-Hour Power Plan (or other plans).

The first days of the routines often recommend squats and deadlifts. Basically, because these are great exercises to learn and master as they can really help you progress quickly with your fitness and fat loss goals. However, they are also big moves that carry some risk if not approached correctly. They may also be too daunting for some.

While I would encourage you to challenge yourself to safely learn all of the exercises included in the routines, there is always flexibility and options, for example:

☑   You can try them first without weight until you feel comfortable you can perform them correctly without risk of injury, then just use a bar or low weight, and build it up from there.

☑ You can interchange with one of the alternative moves from the Alternative Moves table and go back to the original moves later when you feel more comfortable. See the Alternative Moves table on the website: BIT.LY/ALTMOVES

☑ You can do 3 weeks with one move and then a variant on the 4th week to keep things varied and "surprise" the muscles. You could of course change the move every week although chopping and changing this quickly can make it harder to progress with things like strength. A reasonable degree of uniformity and consistency is generally more helpful to progression.

☑ Whenever you're unsure, drop the weight before you try!

☑ Aim for the suggested reps, but drop the weight if necessary. Remember, total volume is often more important than the reps you do each set. So if you go short on one set, drop the weight and up the reps on the next set or vice versa.

THE 3-HOUR POWER PLAN

The Lean Exec approach is to exercise as much as you can within your ability to recover. If you have a busy job and personal life, it can have a major impact on how much you can train. In addition, if you don't sleep well, training can be that extra bit harder. Don't despair, though; with some persistence and resilience you can change that! The 3-Hour Power Plan is a training routine I designed so I could still make progress in the gym during busy periods, in as little as three hours per week. The key things I aimed to achieve with the plan were:

☑ Progress within ability to recover.

☑ Minimal time in the gym without losing intensity.

☑ Comprehensive body coverage to ensure symmetry and balance.

☑ Ability/option to focus training around weekends if necessary.

NOTE: BIGGER BROTHER RECOMMENDS USING THESE BASE EXERCISES. HOWEVER, IF FOR ANY REASON (E.G. EQUIPMENT NOT AVAILABLE, OR SIMPLY FOR VARIATION AFTER A FEW MONTHS) YOU NEED TO CHANGE THE MOVES, SEE THE ALTERNATIVE MOVES TABLE ON THE WEBSITE: BIT.LY/ALTMOVES FOR OPTIONS ON EACH EXERCISE.

Rest Between Exercises

Typical rest times between sets in this training are between 45 and 90 seconds. When transitioning between exercises it's OK to rest a bit longer, although we would encourage you to keep any rest in the gym under 120 seconds, where possible.

SUGGESTED SCHEDULE | WORKOUT PATTERN & BASE EXERCISES REQUIRED

Weekday	1	2	3	4	5	6	7
Workout Pattern 1	1	2	3	Rest	Rest or 4	Rest	Rest
Workout Pattern 2	1	2	Rest	3	Rest or 4	Rest	Rest
Workout Pattern 3	1	Rest	2	3	Rest or 4	Rest	Rest

Day 1 Legs & Core	Day 2 Chest & Back	Day 3 Triceps & Biceps	Day 4 (Optional) Weak Points
Cardio	Cardio	Cardio	Increased Cardio
Back Squat	Pull-Ups	Barbell / EZ-Bar Bicep Curl (Palms Up & Palms Down)	Pull-Ups
Deadlift	Shoulder / Military Press	Tricep Dips	Push-Ups
Leg Curls	Bench Press (+Variations)	Medium Grip or Close Grip Seated Preacher Curls	Body Weight Squats
Calf Raises	Lat Pull-Downs	V-Bar Tricep Push-Down	Weak Points
	Seated Row	Tricep Overhead Extension	

3-HOUR POWER PLAN | DAY 1
Time to complete: 50 minutes – 1 hour

Day 1

No.	Exercise	Set	Minimum Reps	Optimal Target Reps	Estimated % of One Rep Max	Guide Tempo	Rest Period After Set (Seconds)	Training Notes
1	Cardio Warm-Up	1	5–10 Min					This should start slow (e.g. a light jog), but elevate to around 50–70% of your max effort. Ensure you get the blood flowing, but don't overdo it.

Note: You may want to try some static or dynamic stretching. See: Warming Up, Stretching & Cooling Down

No.	Exercise	Set	Minimum Reps	Optimal Target Reps	Estimated % of One Rep Max	Guide Tempo	Rest Period After Set (Seconds)	Training Notes
2	Standard Back Squat							

Note: Barbell squats can cause serious injury if not performed correctly. Ensure you use safety bars and/or a spotter. If in doubt about a weight, go lower first and perform the move with full range of motion and correct form until you are confident you can increase the weight.

Set	Minimum Reps	Optimal Target Reps	Estimated % of One Rep Max	Guide Tempo	Rest Period After Set (Seconds)	Training Notes
1	15	20	0%	2020	60	Warm Up Body Weight Squats.
2	12	15	55%	2010	60-90	Aim for 15, go lighter if necessary.
3	10	12	60%	2010	60-90	The weight should be heavy enough that
4	8	10	60%	2010	60-90	you can't lift more than the optimal target
5	5	8	60%	2010	60-90	reps per set. Optional final set. If you feel good, go for it!
Total Reps	50	65				

3 Deadlift (Or Trap Bar Deadlift)

Note: Deadlifts can cause serious injury to the lower back if not performed correctly. Ensure you use good form and go lower on the weight until you feel comfortable you can perform quality reps with full range of motion.

Set	Reps	Reps	%	Tempo	Rest	
1	10	15	60%	1020	60–90	Aim for 15, go lighter if necessary.
2	10	15	60%	1020	60–90	Concentrate on correct form and control with a heavy, yet manageable weight, over just trying to get the reps done.
Total Reps	20	30				

4 Calf Raise

Set	Reps	Reps	%	Tempo	Rest	
1	15	20	50%	2020	60	Don't go too light, but make sure you can do 15–20 good quality reps.
2	12	15	60%	2020	60–90	
3	10	12	70%	2020	60–90	Ensure you stretch and tense and pump the calves 5–10 times after each set.
4	10	12	70%	2020	60–90	
Total Reps	47	59				

5 Leg Curl (Optional: Recovering well? Try adding this to the workout)

Type	Set	Reps	Reps	%	Tempo	Rest	
Seated	1	15	20	50%	1212	60	Don't go too light, but make sure you can do 15–20 good quality reps.
or	2	12	15	60%	1212	60–90	
Lying	3	10	12	70%	1212	60–90	If you're progressing well, try adding this to the workout to see how your body responds. If it feels OK, keep going.
	4	10	12	70%	1212	60–90	
Total Reps		47	59				

6 Cardio Warm-Down

Set	Time	
1	10-15 Min	Run, bike, skate, whatever you like, just get the blood pumping. You should already be sweating from the training, but don't stop, go fast, go intense, try intervals, finish your workout with pride!

Note: It's recommended that you include a 3–5 minute low-intensity cool down.

Day 2

No.	Exercise	Set	Minimum Reps	Optimal Target Reps	Estimated % of One Rep Max	Guide Tempo	Rest Period After Set (Seconds)	Training Notes
1	Cardio Warm-Up							This should start slow (e.g. a light jog), but elevate to around 50–70% of your max effort. Ensure you get the blood flowing, but don't overdo it.
		1	5–10 Min					
	Note: You may want to try some static or dynamic stretching. See: Warming Up, Stretching & Cooling Down							
2	Pull-Ups							
		1	To Failure	15	N/A	1010	60–90	Do as many as you can for each set.
		2	To Failure	10	N/A	1010	60–90	If you can't do any (or any more), do negative reps to failure. This will help increase your strength and, if you keep it up your pull-up strength will improve.
		3	To Failure	10	N/A	1010	60–90	
		4	To Failure	10	N/A	1010	60–90	
	Total Reps		24	45				
3	Shoulder Press	Seated or Standing (Military Press)						
		1	8	10	75%	1020	60–90	
		2	8	10	75%	1020	60–90	
		3	8	10	65%	1020	60–90	
		4	To Failure	To Failure	50%	1020		Only do this final set if you were not failing on the final reps of set 3–4.
	Total Reps		24	30				
4	Incline Bench Press	Medium Grip (Try Close & Wide Grip Some Weeks)						
		1	8	10	70%	1020	60–90	This should be heavy enough that you can only just lift 3–4 reps, no more.
		2	3	4	80%	1020	60–90	
		3	8	10	65%	1020	45–60	
		4	6	10	50%	1020		This is a drop set, so you can keep going until failure.
	Total Reps		25	34				

5 Lat Pull-Down | Wide Grip (Try Close/Hammer Grip Some Weeks)

1	10	12	65%	1020	60-90	This should be heavy enough that you can only lift the reps, no more.
2	3	6	85%	1020	60-90	
3	4	6	75%	1020	45-60	This is a drop set, so you can keep going until failure.
4	8	10	50%	1020		
Total Reps	25	34				

6 Flat (or 1 level Incline) Bench Press

1	10	12	65%	1020	60-90
2	6	8	80%	1020	60-90
3	8	10	75%	1020	45-60
4	To Failure	To Failure	50%	1020		Only do this final set if you were not failing on the final reps of set 2–3.
Total Reps	24	30			

7 Hammer Grip Seated Row (Machine or Cable)

1	10	12	65%	1020	60-90
2	8	10	80%	1020	60-90	You can also try wide grip rows some weeks.
3	8	10	65%	1020	45-60
Total Reps	26	32			

6 Cardio Warm-Down

1   10-15 Min

Note: It's recommended that you include a 3–5 minute low-intensity cool down.

Run, bike, skate, whatever you like, just get the blood pumping. You should already be sweating from the training, but don't stop, go fast, go intense, try intervals, finish your workout with pride!

3-HOUR POWER PLAN | DAY 3
Time to complete: 50 minutes – 1 hour

Day 3

No.	Exercise	Set	Minimum Reps	Optimal Target Reps	Estimated % of One Rep Max	Guide Tempo	Rest Period After Set (Seconds)	Training Notes
1	Cardio Warm-Up							This should start slow (e.g. a light jog), but elevate to around 50–70% of your max effort. Ensure you get the blood flowing, but don't overdo it.
		1	5–10 Min					

Note: You may want to try some static or dynamic stretching. See: Warming Up, Stretching & Cooling Down

No.	Exercise	Set	Minimum Reps	Optimal Target Reps	Estimated % of One Rep Max	Guide Tempo	Rest Period After Set (Seconds)	Training Notes
2A	Standard Grip (Palms Up/Supination) Ez-Bar Bicep Curl							
		1	15	20	Bar Only	1010	60–90	Warm Up.
		2	8	10	70%	1120	60–90	
		3	2	4	80%	1120	60–90	Choose a challenging weight, but make sure you use correct form.
		4	8	10	70%	1120	60–90	
	Total Reps		33	44				
2B	Switch To: Reverse Grip (Palms Down) Ez-Bar Bicep Curl							
		5	8	10	65%	1020	60–90	Reverse Grip Curls are usually harder than palms up curls so you may need to drop the weight.
		6	8	10	65%	1020	60–90	
		7	8	12	50%	1020	60–90	This is a drop set, so you can keep going until failure.
	Total Reps		24	32				

3 Tricep Dips (Body Weight)

Set	Target	Reps	%	Tempo	Rest	Notes
1	To Failure	15	N/A	1010	60–90	*Do as many as you can for each set.*
2	To Failure	10	N/A	1010	60–90	*If you can't do any (or any more), do negative reps to failure. This will help increase your strength, and if you keep it up, your Dip strength will improve.*
3	To Failure	10	N/A	1010	60–90	
4	To Failure	10	N/A	1010	60–90	
Total Reps		45				

4A Medium (V-Bar) Grip Triceps (Palms Down/Pronation) Push-down

Set	Reps	Reps	%	Tempo	Rest	Notes
1	12	15	50%	1010	60–90	*Warm Up.*
2	8	10	70%	1120	60–90	
3	2	4	80%	1120	60–90	*Choose a challenging weight, but make sure you use correct form.*
4	8	10	70%	1120	60–90	
Total Reps	30	39				

4B Switch To: Tricep Overhead Extension with Rope

Set	Reps	Reps	%	Tempo	Rest	Notes
5	8	10	65%	1020	60–90	*Use a challenging weight you can lift with good form.*
6	8	10	65%	1020	45–60	
7	8	12	50%	1020		*This is a drop set, so you can keep going until failure.*
Total Reps	24	32				

5 Cardio Warm-Down

Set	Time	Notes
1	10–15 Min	*Run, bike, skate, whatever you like, just get the blood pumping. You should already be sweating from the training, but don't stop. go fast, go intense, try intervals, finish your workout with pride!*

Note: It's recommended that you include a 3–5 min low-intensity cool down.

3-HOUR POWER PLAN | DAY 4 (OPTIONAL)
Time to complete: 45 minutes – 1 Hour

Day 4 (Optional)

No.	Exercise	Set	Minimum Reps	Optimal Target Reps	Estimated % of One Rep Max	Guide Tempo	Rest Period After Set (Seconds)	Training Notes
1	Cardio Warm-Up	1	5–10 Min					This should start slow (e.g. a light jog), but elevate to around 50–70% of your max effort. Ensure you get the blood flowing, but don't overdo it.

Note: You may want to try some static or dynamic stretching. See: Warming Up, Stretching & Cooling Down

No.	Exercise	Set	Minimum Reps	Optimal Target Reps	Estimated % of One Rep Max	Guide Tempo	Rest Period After Set (Seconds)	Training Notes
2	Pull-Ups	1	Max	Max	Bodyweight	1010	60–75	Target 1: 20 Reps Total
		2	Max	Max	Bodyweight	1010	60–75	Target 2: 30 Reps Total
		3	Max	Max	Bodyweight	1010	60–75	Target 3: 40 Reps Total
		4	Max	Max	Bodyweight	1010	60–75	Target 4: 50 Reps Total
		5	Max	Max	Bodyweight	1010		Note: These are long-term targets. Mix it up with a 2020 tempo.

3 Push-Ups (Try close grip if you want more focus on your Triceps)

1	Max	Bodyweight	1010	60–75	Target 1: 25 Reps Total
2	Max	Bodyweight	1010	60–75	Target 2: 50 Reps Total
3	Max	Bodyweight	1010	60–75	Target 3: 75 Reps Total
4	Max	Bodyweight	1010	60–75	Target 4: 100 Reps Total
5	Max	Bodyweight	1010		Note: These are long-term targets. Mix it up with a 2020 tempo.

4 Body Weight Squats (Or choose a lower body weak point, e.g. Calves)

1	10	20	Bodyweight	1010	60–75	Try different tempos. Sometimes you can go quickly doing 1010 and other times you can slow it right down to 2222. The latter will be harder so you may not do as many reps, but it will help you get stronger.
2	10	20	Bodyweight	1010	60–75
3	10	20	Bodyweight	1010	60–75
4	10	20	Bodyweight	1010	60–75
5	0	20	Bodyweight	1010	

Total Reps 40 100

5 Cardio Warm-Down

1 20–30 Min

Note: It's recommended that you include a 3–5 min low-intensity cool down.

Run, bike, skate, whatever you like, just get the blood pumping. You should already be sweating from the training, but don't stop, go fast, go intense, try intervals, finish your workout with pride!

FOR WEEKS WHEN YOU HAVE THAT EXTRA HOUR OR TWO

The Lean Exec training is designed to be flexible and take advantage of the fact that change is good and can be the catalyst that fuels progress in the gym and in life. Even for the busiest people, there are always those weeks when you have a bit more time than usual. These times are great for pushing progress! A fourth day is included in this plan, which is recommended if you can fit it into your schedule.

PUMP IT UP! TRAINING PLAN

For when you have more time on your hands, you're sleeping well, you're eating well, you've got plenty of energy and really want to maximise your progress in the gym. Hey, you've even got the craving to go to the gym on your rest day – you're looking for your rest muscle and wondering how you can train it! This plan is for those times when you're super-motivated and can find the time to train well, 5–6 times a week.

This is a similarly balanced plan for the weekly training, but requires more regular trips to the gym. This training is based on foundation training I did to gain 20kg of muscle size and strength when I was at university (all those years ago) and adapted in recent years. Please ensure you complete the exercises with the correct form (as described earlier in this book) and follow the plan as closely as possible for maximum results. It's important to note (again) that nutrition also plays a vital role in progress. Optimising your diet based on the nutrition suggestions in this book and on The Lean Exec website will ensure you have the best opportunity of making significant progress in the short-est space of time.

Pump Importance!

Unless you are in great fitness, eating and sleeping really well, this plan can be hard for busy people (depend-ing on your age, sleep quality and fitness level). Make sure you are getting plenty of rest and eating the right volume of the correct macronutrient calories. As this plan works different body parts on different days, make sure you are working at similar levels for each of the days or you can get body part lag and less balanced development. Listen to your body, keep it flexible, but, if you are struggling to complete the first four days of this plan with equal vigour, it's best to switch back to the 3-Hour Power Plan then add in the Pump It Up! Plan days 5 and 6 if/where possible.

SUGGESTED SCHEDULE | WORKOUT PATTERN & BASE EXERCISES REQUIRED

Weekday	1	2	3	4	5	6	7
Workout Pattern Option 1	1	2	3	4	5	Rest or 6	Rest
Workout Pattern Option 2	1	2	Rest	3	4	5	Rest

Day 1 Legs & Core	Day 2 Chest & Triceps	Day 3 Back & Biceps	Day 4 Shoulders	Day 5 Weak Points	Day 6 Active Rest
Cardio	Cardio	Cardio	Increased Cardio	Various	Ab Crunches
Back Squat	Push-Ups	Pull-Ups	Shoulder Press		The Plank
Deadlift	Bench Press (+Variations)	Hammer Grip Seated Rows	Side Lateral Raise		Upward Dog
Leg Curls	Dips	Lat Pull-Downs (+Variations)	Machine Flys / Reverse Flys		Child Restful Pose
Calf Raises	Tricep Push-Downs	Bicep Curls			Cardio
	Tricep Extension	Machine Rows			

NOTE: BIGGER BROTHER RECOMMENDS USING THESE BASE EXERCISES. HOWEVER, IF FOR ANY REASON (E.G. EQUIPMENT NOT AVAILABLE, OR SIMPLY FOR VARIATION AFTER 6 WEEKS OR MORE) YOU NEED TO CHANGE THE MOVES, SEE THE ALTERNATIVE MOVES TABLE ON THE WEBSITE: BIT.LY/ALTMOVES FOR OPTIONS ON EACH EXERCISE.

Rest Between Exercises

Typical rest times between sets in this training are between 45 and 90 seconds. When transitioning between exercises, it's OK to rest a bit longer, although we would encourage you to keep any rest in the gym under 120 seconds, where possible.

PUMP IT UP! PLAN | DAY 1 – CORE & LEGS
Time to complete: aim for under 1 hour, max 1 hour 10 minutes [70 minutes].

Day 1

No.	Exercise	Set	Minimum Reps	Optimal Target Reps	Estimated % of One Rep Max	Guide Tempo	Rest Period After Set (Seconds)	Training Notes
1	Cardio Warm-Up							This should start slow (e.g. a light jog), but elevate to around 50–70% of your max effort. Ensure you get the blood flowing, but don't overdo it.
		1	5–10 Min					
	Note: You may want to try some static or dynamic stretching. See: Warming Up, Stretching & Cooling Down							
2	Standard Back Squat							
	Note: Barbell squats can cause serious injury if not performed correctly. Ensure you use safety bars and/or a spotter. If in doubt about a weight, go lower first and perform the move with full range of motion and correct form until you are confident you can increase the weight.							
		1	15	20	0%	1010	60	Warm Up Body Weight Squats.
		2	10	15	55%	2010	60–110	Aim for 15, go lighter if necessary.
		3	8	10	70%	2010	60–110	The weight should be heavy enough that you can't lift more than the optimal target reps.
		4	8	10	70%	2010	60–110	
		5	8	10	55%	2010	60–110	
	Total Reps		49	65				
3	Deadlift (Or Trap Deadlift)							
	Note: Deadlifts can cause serious injury to the lower back if not performed correctly. Ensure you use good form and go lower on the weight until you feel comfortable you can perform quality reps with full range of motion. Concentrate on correct form and control, with a heavy yet manageable weight, over just trying to get the reps done.							
		1	8	12	60%	1020	60–90	Aim for 15, go lighter if necessary.
		2	8	12	60%	1020	60–90	Listen to your body. If the last set feels too much, drop the weight or leave it a week. Although don't cheat yourself, push it and focus on some good nutrition and recovery!
		3	8	12	60%	1020	60–90	
		4	Optional Further Set					
	Total Reps		24	36				

4 Leg Curl (Seated or Lying)

Set					Notes
1	15	20	50%	2020	60	Don't go too light, but make sure you can do 15–20 good quality reps.
2	15	18	60%	2020	60–90	
3	12	15	70%	2020	60–90	
4	10	10	70%	2020	60–90	
5	8	10	60%	2020		
Total Reps	60	73				

5 Calf Raise

Set					Notes
1	15	20	50%	1212	60	Don't go too light, but make sure you can do 15–20 good quality reps.
2	15	18	60%	1212	60–90	
3	12	15	70%	1212	60–90	Ensure you stretch, tense and pump the calves 5–10 times after each set.
4	10	10	70%	1212	60–90	
5	8	10	60%	1212	60–90	
Total Reps	60	73				

6 Cardio Warm-Down

Set		Notes
1	10–15 Min	Run, bike, skate, whatever you like, just get the blood pumping. You should already be sweating from the training, but don't stop, go fast, go intense, try intervals, finish your workout with pride!

Note: It's recommended that you include a 3–5 minute low-intensity cool down.

PUMP IT UP! PLAN | DAY 2 – CHEST & TRICEPS
Time to complete: aim for under 1 hour

Day 2

No.	Exercise	Set	Minimum Reps	Optimal Target Reps	Estimated % of One Rep Max	Guide Tempo	Rest Period After Set (Seconds)	Training Notes
1	Cardio Warm-Up							This should start slow (e.g. a light jog), but elevate to around 50–70% of your max effort. Ensure you get the blood flowing, but don't overdo it.
		1	5–10 Min					
	Note: You may want to try some static or dynamic stretching. See: Warming Up, Stretching & Cooling Down							
2	Push-Ups							*If you can't do Push-Ups, don't give up. See the section: SIU Principle*
		1	To Failure	10+	N/A	1111	60–90	
		2	To Failure	10+	N/A	1111	60–90	Do as many as you can for each set.
		3	To Failure	10+	N/A	1111	60–90	*If you can't do any (or any more), try resting for 10–15 seconds, then trying another 1-2*
		4	To Failure	10+	N/A	1111	60–90	*(or even half) reps.*
	Total Reps			40+				
3	Close Grip Incline Bench Press (2 Weeks Barbell, 1 Week Switch To Dumbbells)							
		1	15	20	Bar Only	1010	60–90	
		2	9	10	65%	1121	60–90	
		3	2	3	90%	1121	60–90	This should be heavy enough that you can only just lift 3 reps, no more.
		4	2	3	85%	1121	45–60	
		5	6	8	70%	1110		*Optional: Do this drop set if you don't feel that you maxed out on sets 3 and 4.*
	Total Reps		34	44				

4 Standard Flat Bench Press (2 Weeks Barbell, 1 Week Switch To Dumbbells)

Set	Reps	Reps	Weight	Tempo	Rest	Notes
1	15	20	Bar Only	1121	60-90	*This should be heavy enough that you can only just lift 3-4 reps, no more.*
2	9	10	65%	1121	60-90	
3	2	3	90%	1121	45-60	
4	7	10	65%	1110	60-90	*This is a drop set, so you can keep going until failure.*
Total Reps	33	43				

5 Tricep Dips (Body Weight)

Set	Reps	Reps	Weight	Tempo	Rest	Notes
1	To Failure	10+	N/A	1020	60-90	*If you can't do any (or any more), try resting for 10-15 seconds, then doing another 1-2 reps. Also try negative reps, using your legs to push yourself into the straight arm position and lowering yourself down.*
2	To Failure	10+	N/A	1020	60-90	
3	To Failure	10+	N/A	1020	60-90	
Total Reps	30+					

6A Medium (V-Bar or Straight bar) Grip Triceps (Palms Down/Pronation) Push-Down

Set	Reps	Reps	Weight	Tempo	Rest	Notes
1	15	20	Bar Only	1010	60-90	*Warm Up.*
2	8	10	70%	1120	60-90	
3	2	3	85%	1120	60-90	*Choose a challenging weight, but make sure you use correct form.*
4	3	4	80%	1120	60-90	
Total Reps	28	37				

6B Switch To: Tricep Overhead Extension with Rope

Set	Reps	Reps	Weight	Tempo	Rest	Notes
5	6	8	75%	1020	60-90	
6	8	10	70%	1020	60-90	
7	8	12	50%	1020	45-60	*This is a drop set, so you can keep going until failure.*
Total Reps	22	30				

7 Cardio Warm-Down

Set	Duration	Notes
1	5-10 Min	*Run, bike, skate, whatever you like, just get the blood pumping. You should already be sweating from the training, but don't stop, go fast, go intense, try intervals, finish your workout with pride!*

Note: It's recommended that you include a 3-5 minute low-intensity cool down.

Day 3

No.	Exercise	Set	Minimum Reps	Optimal Target Reps	Estimated % of One Rep Max	Guide Tempo	Rest Period After Set (Seconds)	Training Notes
1	Cardio Warm-Up							
		1	5–10 Min					This should start slow (e.g. a light jog), but elevate to around 50–70% of your max effort. Ensure you get the blood flowing, but don't overdo it.
	Note: You may want to try some static or dynamic stretching. See: Warming Up, Stretching & Cooling Down							
2	Pull-Ups							If you can't do Pull-Ups, don't give up. See the section: SIU Principle
		1	To Failure	15	N/A	1020	60–75	Do as many as you can for each set.
		2	To Failure	10	N/A	1020	60–90	If you can't do any (or any more), try resting for 15 sec, then doing 1–2 reps.
		3	To Failure	5	N/A	1020	60–90	
		4	To Failure	5	N/A	1020	45	
		5	To Failure	5	N/A	1020	45	If you can't do any (or anymore), do negative reps to failure. This will help increase your strength and if you keep it up your Pull-Up strength will improve.
		6	To Failure	5	N/A	1030	45	
		7	To Failure	5	N/A	1030	45	
	Total Reps			50				
3	Hammer Grip Seated Row (Machine or Cable)							
		1	10	12	65%	1020	60–90	
		2	8	10	80%	1020	60–90	
		3	8	10	75%	1020	45–60	
		4	To Failure	To Failure	50%	1020		Only do this final set if you were not failing on the final reps of set 2–3.
	Total Reps		26	32				

4 Wide Grip Lat Pull Down (Medium Grip is OK, but go wide if possible)

Set	Reps	Reps	%	Tempo	Rest	Notes
1	10	12	65%	1020	60-90	
2	8	10	80%	1020	60-90	
3	8	10	75%	1020	45-60	
4	To Failure	To Failure	50%	1020	60-90	Only do this final set if you were not failing on the final reps of set 2-3.
Total Reps	26	32				

5A Wide Grip (Palms Up/Supination) Ez-Bar Bicep Curl

Set	Reps	Reps	%	Tempo	Rest	Notes
1	15	20	Bar Only	1010	60-90	Warm Up.
2	8	10	70%	1120	60-90	
3	2	2	85%	1120	60-90	Choose a challenging weight, but make sure you use correct form.
4	2	2	85%	1120	60-90	
Total Reps	27	35				

5B Switch To: Reverse Grip (Palms Down) Ez-Bar Bicep Curl

Set	Reps	Reps	%	Tempo	Rest	Notes
5	5	5	75%	1020	60-90	Reverse Grip Curls are usually harder than Palms Up Curls so you may need to drop the weight.
6	8	10	70%	1020	60-90	
7	8	12	50%	1020	60-90	This is a drop set, so you can keep going until failure.
Total Reps	21	27				

6 Wide Grip Machine Rows

Set	Reps	Reps	%	Tempo	Rest	Notes
1	12	15	65%	1020	60-90	
2	12	15	65%	1020	60-90	
3	To Failure	To Failure	50%	1020		
Total Reps	24	30				If you're feeling good, repeat sets 2 and 3.

7 Cardio Warm-Down

Set	Time	Notes
1	5-10 Min	Run, bike, skate, whatever you like, just get the blood pumping. You should already be sweating from the training, but don't stop, go fast, go intense, try intervals, finish your workout with pride!

Note: It's recommended that you include a 3-5 minute low-intensity cool down.

Day 4

No.	Exercise	Set	Minimum Reps	Optimal Target Reps	Estimated % of One Rep Max	Guide Tempo	Rest Period After Set (Seconds)	Training Notes
1	Cardio Warm-Up							This should start slow (e.g. a light jog), but elevate to around 50–70% of your max effort. Ensure you get the blood flowing, but don't overdo it.
		1	5–10 Min					

Note: You may want to try some static or dynamic stretching. See: Warming Up, Stretching & Cooling Down

No.	Exercise	Set	Minimum Reps	Optimal Target Reps	Estimated % of One Rep Max	Guide Tempo	Rest Period After Set (Seconds)	Training Notes
2	Dumbbell Shoulder Press	Seated or Standing (Military Press)						
		1	8	12	80%	2020	60–90	Try using a barbell some weeks.
		2	8	10	80%	2020	60–90	
		3	8	10	65%	2020	60–90	
		4	6	8	65%	2020	45–60	
		5	To Failure	To Failure	50%	2020		Only do this final set if you were not failing on the final reps of set 3–4.
	Total Reps		30	40				

3 Dumbbell Side Lateral Raise

Set					
1	8	12	65%	1110	60–90
2	8	10	60%	1110	60–90
3	6	8	50%	1110	60–90
4	6	8	65%	1110	45–60
5	To Failure	To Failure	50%	1110	
Total Reps	28	38			

Make sure you use good control when lifting the weights. Imagine the dumbbells are glasses filled with water and tip some of the water out at the top of the move (arms fully raised at shoulder height).

This is a drop set, so you can keep going until failure.

4 Machine (Chest!?) Flys (MF) Vs Reverse Flys (RF)

	Set					
MF	1	12	15	50%	1010	60–90
RF	2	12	15	50%	1010	60–90
MF	3	12	15	50%	1010	60–90
RF	4	12	15	50%	1010	45–60
Total Reps	48	60				

Machine Flys are technically a chest move, but Bigger Brother likes to do these for a 360-degree finish. It's the Symmitarian way! Alternate between front and reverse flys with relatively light weight, high reps and low rest between alternations. Go wide and back for a nice chest stretch.

5 Cardio Warm-Down

1	5–10 Min	

Note: It's recommended that you include a 3–5 minute low-intensity cool down.

Run, bike, skate, whatever you like, just get the blood pumping. You should already be sweating from the training, but don't stop, go fast, go intense, try intervals, finish your workout with pride!

Day 5

No.	Exercise	Set	Minimum Reps	Optimal Target Reps	Estimated % of One Rep Max	Guide Tempo	Rest Period After Set (Seconds)	Training Notes
1	Cardio Warm-Up							This should start slow (e.g. a light jog), but elevate to around 50–70% of your max effort. Ensure you get the blood flowing, but don't overdo it.
		1	5–10 Min					

Note: You may want to try some static or dynamic stretching. See: Warming Up, Stretching & Cooling Down

2 Lower Body | Legs

Example: Calf Raise | Leg Curl. If you are doing your Core & Legs day properly you should not feel the need to do quads or moves like squats or deadlifts that hit your lower back. In any case, you may be best advised to avoid squats and deadlifts more than once per week until you are very advanced.

No.	Exercise	Set	Minimum Reps	Optimal Target Reps	Estimated % of One Rep Max	Guide Tempo	Rest Period After Set (Seconds)	Training Notes
		1	15	20	50%	1212	60–90	Don't go too light, but make sure you can do
		2	10	15	70%	1212	60–90	15–20 good quality reps.
		3	10	15	70%	1212	60–90	Ensure you stretch and tense the calves.
		4	10	15	60%	1212	45–60	
		5	To Failure	To Failure	50%	1010		This is a drop set, so you can keep going until failure.
	Total Reps		45	65				

3 Upper Body

Example: Bicep Curls | Tricep Push-Downs. As with legs, focus on smaller muscle groups that are lagging or feel less trained that week. Avoid big lifts that put pressure on your lower back.

					Notes
1	10	12	65%	1020	60-90	Don't go too light, but make sure you can do 10-12 good quality reps. Ensure you stretch and tense the muscle.
2	8	10	60%	1020	60-90
3	6	8	60%	1020	60-90
4	8	10	50%	1020	45-60
5	To Failure	To Failure	50%	1010	This is a drop set, so you can keep going until failure.
Total Reps	32	40			

4+ Do 1 or 2 complementary moves for the following sets

					Notes
1	8	12	50%	1020	60-90	Listen to your body. Do the extra moves if you feel you don't have complete body coverage. You should find it reasonably difficult to finish the final rep. If not, it may be time to increase the weight.
2	8	12	50%	1020	60-90
3	8	10	50%	1020	60-90
4	To Failure	To Failure	50%	1020	45-60

5 Cardio Warm-Down

1	5–10 Min	Run, bike, skate, whatever you like, just get the blood pumping. You should already be sweating from the training, but don't stop, go fast, go intense, try intervals, finish your workout with pride!

Note: It's recommended that you include a 3–5 minute low-intensity cool down.

Day 6

Note: You may want to try some static or dynamic stretching. See: Warming Up, Stretching & Cooling Down

1 Ab Crunches (Or Hanging Leg Raises)

No.	Exercise	Set	Minimum Reps	Optimal Target Reps	Estimated % of One Rep Max	Guide Tempo	Rest Period After Set (Seconds)	Training Notes
		1	20	25	Bodyweight	1010	60–90	Don't clasp hands around head.
		2	20	25	Bodyweight	1010	60–90	Keep fingertips lightly touching the temples/side of head.
		3	20	25	Bodyweight	1010	60–90	
		4	20	25	Bodyweight	1010	45–60	Focus on a tight movement, controlled tensing of the abs. Don't use momentum.
		5	Max	Max	Bodyweight	1010		
	Total Reps		80	100				

2 The Plank

	Hold For:	Set	Seconds	Seconds	Estimated % of One Rep Max	Guide Tempo	Rest Period After Set (Seconds)	Training Notes
		1	20	30	Bodyweight	N/A	45–60	Focus on control and form. Have patience, improvements will come.
		2	20	30	Bodyweight	N/A	45–60	Target 1: 4x 30 sec holds
		3	20	30	Bodyweight	N/A	45–60	Target 2: 4x 45 sec holds
		4	20	30	Bodyweight	N/A	46–60	Target 3: 4x 60 sec holds
		5	Max	Max	Bodyweight	N/A		Target 4: 1x 90 sec hold
								Target 5: 1x 2 min hold
								Don't give up too easy!

3 Upward Dog

Hold For:

	Seconds	Seconds			
1	10	30	Bodyweight	N/A	45-60
2	10	30	Bodyweight	N/A	45-60
3	10	30	Bodyweight	N/A	45-60
4	10	30	Bodyweight	N/A	45-60
5	Max	Max	Bodyweight	N/A	

Concentrate on keeping your waist on or close to the floor. Put your chin high and look up. Ensure a gentle stretch of the lower back. It's OK to have slightly bent arms, but try to work your way towards fully straight arms with each workout.

4 Child Restful Pose

Hold For:

	Seconds	Seconds			
1	10	15	Bodyweight	N/A	45-60
2	10	15	Bodyweight	N/A	45-60
3	10	15	Bodyweight	N/A	45-60
4	10	15	Bodyweight	N/A	

Try experimenting with different hold times and repeat the pose a few times each session, if you wish.

5 Cardio Warm-Down

1	5-10 Min

Note: It's recommended that you include a 3-5 minute low-intensity cool down.

Run, bike, skate, whatever you like, just get the blood pumping. You should already be sweating from the training, but don't stop, go fast, go intense, try intervals, finish your workout with pride!

AVOIDING & BREAKING PLATEAUS

If you are someone who is new to training, following the plans and keeping your diet and sleep in reasonable order, you will see progress and limited plateaus at least in the first 6 weeks to three months. In principle, as long as you are progressively overloading within your training, you do not have to change the basis of your workout until you reach a size and weight that you are happy with long-term.

However, there are always times when things can feel like they have hit a block and are not moving as quickly as they have done before. You can use some of the "plateau-busting" techniques described throughout this book to ensure you are continually advancing. Ultimately, results will come with a combination of consistency in your training, eating and rest. However, it's understandable that doing the same things, week in and week out, can become boring and affect motivation. If you want to alter your training to keep it interesting, look at the alternative and substitute moves you can do in the Alternative Moves part of the website.

If you've been training for six weeks or more and feel like you have either stopped advancing or are lacking motivation, it can help to take a week off. Continue to eat well (and by eat well, I mean good nutritional food) during that week and do light exercise, like walking and stretching. You can also try low-intensity exercise, like yoga. Some people worry that taking a week off (even when sick) will slow down their progress and they will lose the muscle gains. While you might find a small drop on your first few sessions back after a break, if you have continued to eat right you are likely to find that you quickly regain that strength and likely surpass it by week two. In reality, rest and recuperation periods can be advantageous in terms of breaking plateaus and regaining motivation for another gym stretch. Endlessly battering your body and/or doing "lazy workouts" due to boredom/lack of motivation can have negative effects. However, that's not to say you should be lazy and take long periods off! Here are some Bigger Brother suggestions for breaking plateaus, maintaining motivation and keeping your mental fitness focused on the goal.

☑ Try to set yourself regular long- and short-term goals. This can be as simple as, "I will add 2kg to my deadlift each week until I reach my target" or "I need to stick to my routine for the next two months so I'm ready for the beach". The key thing is – set goals and break them down into small steps.

☑ Try another gym, or better yet, train with a friend at their gym. Most gyms offer free passes and discount rates for a trial day. The change in scenery can give your workout that extra boost.

☑ Train with a partner. Training with a partner can help push you on days when you're not feeling that inspired.

☑ Take a week off. Although, as mentioned above, this should be following a reasonable stretch of training and not be for more than a week or so. This can help you recalibrate for another stretch. Also, you could try active breaks. This could be as simple as doing one to two weeks of the conditioning programme again, to your max intensity. (If you've been doing the foundation training for a while, you should get a boost from the difference in your level when re-engaging in the conditioning training.) Alternatively, go snowboarding, surfing, kayaking, or whatever physical sport/ adventure excites you for an active break from the gym.

☑ Do your training for one or two weeks using slightly lower weight and increased reps. For example, if you usually do 50kg for 5–6 reps on your first set, do 40–45kg for 7–8 reps. The slight change and feeling of the lighter weight can sometimes make you feel good and the variation may even help break a plateau.

☑ Assuming you're already warmed up, start your sets for a move lifting pretty near your one rep max, if not your actual one rep max. One set like this will not only provide some extra load stimulation, but it can also make the following sets with a usual weight seem slightly lighter than usual.

- ☑ Do a lighter drop set than usual. If your drop set is usually 10kg less, drop it 15–20kg and do reps until failure.

- ☑ Use the alternative (substitute) exercises shown in the plan instead of the main exercises, to add variety. However, try to avoid deviating from the core moves where possible. See the Alternative Moves table on the website: BIT.LY/ALTMOVES

PLATEAU BREAKER TRAINING PLAN

The Plateau Breaker is exactly what it says on the tin! It's designed to help you break a plateau and, in particular, push up your strength. Even if you're not aiming to get big, pushing up your strength will help your training advance. I use this three-hours-a-week training plan, with plenty of good food and rest, to accelerate forward. You could do this training for a number of weeks, but it works well for one or two weeks before returning to the more rounded plans.

SUGGESTED SCHEDULE | WORKOUT PATTERN & BASE EXERCISES REQUIRED

Day 1 Legs & Core	Day 2 Chest, Shoulders & Triceps	Day 3 Back & Biceps
Cardio	Cardio	Cardio
Back Squat	Push-Ups	Pull-Ups
Deadlift	Tricep Dips	Resistance Machine Pull-Ups
	Shoulder/Military Press	Lat Pull-Down
	Bench Press Variations	EZ-Bar Bicep Curls
	Tricep Push-Downs	Seated Rows

Weekday	1	2	3	4	5	6	7
Workout Pattern 1	1	Rest	2	Rest	3	Rest	Rest
Workout Pattern 2	1	2	Rest	3	Rest	Rest	Rest
Workout Pattern 3	1	Rest	2	3	Rest	Rest	Rest

NOTE: BIGGER BROTHER RECOMMENDS USING THESE BASE EXERCISES. HOWEVER, IF FOR ANY REASON (E.G. EQUIPMENT NOT AVAILABLE, OR SIMPLY FOR VARIATION AFTER A FEW MONTHS) YOU NEED TO CHANGE THE MOVES, SEE THE ALTERNATIVE MOVES TABLE ON THE WEBSITE: BIT.LY/ALTMOVES FOR OPTIONS ON EACH EXERCISE.

Rest Between Exercises

Typical rest times between sets in this training are between 45 and 90 seconds. For the Plateau Breaker it's OK to take longer rest times between sets, particularly on Day 1. However, try to keep it as close to 120 seconds as possible, and drop the weight, if necessary. Note, though it should be hard!

PLATEAU BREAKER PLAN | DAY 1
Time to complete: aim for under 1 hour, max 1 hour 10 minutes [70 minutes] including warm up and cool down.

Day 1

No.	Exercise	Set	Minimum Reps	Optimal Target Reps	Estimated % of One Rep Max	Guide Tempo	Rest Period After Set (Seconds)	Training Notes
1	Cardio Warm-Up							
		1	5–10 Min					This should start slow (e.g. a light jog), but elevate to around 50–70% of your max effort. Ensure you get the blood flowing, but don't overdo it.

Note: You may want to try some static or dynamic stretching. See: Warming Up, Stretching & Cooling Down

No.	Exercise	Set	Minimum Reps	Optimal Target Reps	Estimated % of One Rep Max	Guide Tempo	Rest Period After Set (Seconds)	Training Notes
2	Standard Back Squat							

Note: Barbell squats can cause serious injury if not performed correctly. Ensure you use safety bars and/or a spotter. If in doubt about a weight, go lower first and perform the move with full range of motion and correct form until you are confident you can increase the weight.

Set	Minimum Reps	Optimal Target Reps	Estimated % of One Rep Max	Guide Tempo	Rest Period After Set (Seconds)	Training Notes
1	18	20	0%	1010	60	Warm-Up Body Weight Squats (or with bar).
2	12	15	70%	2010	60–110	Choose weight where you can do no more
3	8	10	75%	2010	60–110	than the max reps. Concentrate on correct
4	8	10	80%	2010	60–120	form, tempo and control, over just trying to
5	8	10	80%	2010	60–120	get the reps done.
6	8	10	75%	2010	60–120	
7	8	12	60%	2010		If you've done this correctly, the last reps should be very hard.
Total Reps	70	87				

3 Deadlift

Note: Deadlifts can cause serious injury to the lower back if not performed correctly. Ensure you use good form and go lower on the weight until you feel comfortable you can perform quality reps with full range of motion. Concentrate on correct form and control, with a heavy yet manageable weight, over just trying to get the reps done.

1	10	15	60%	1020	60–110	Aim for 15, go lighter if necessary.
2	10	12	70%	1020	60–110	Weight should be heavy enough that you
3	3	5	80%	1020	60–120	can't lift more than the optimal target reps.
4	8	10	70%	1020	60–120	If you've done this correctly, the last reps
5	8	10	70%	1020		should be very hard.
Total Reps	39	52				If you feel you need it.

4 Cardio Warm-Down

1	10–15 Min

Run, bike, skate, whatever you like, just get the blood pumping. You should already be sweating from the training, but don't stop, go fast, go intense, try intervals, finish your workout with pride!

Note: It's recommended that you include a 3–5 minute low-intensity cool down.

Day 2

No.	Exercise	Set	Minimum Reps	Optimal Target Reps	Estimated % of One Rep Max	Guide Tempo	Rest Period After Set (Seconds)	Training Notes
1	Cardio Warm-Up							
		1	5–10 Min					This should start slow (e.g. a light jog), but elevate to around 50–70% of your max effort. Ensure you get the blood flowing, but don't overdo it.

Note: You may want to try some static or dynamic stretching. See: Warming Up, Stretching & Cooling Down

No.	Exercise	Set	Minimum Reps	Optimal Target Reps	Estimated % of One Rep Max	Guide Tempo	Rest Period After Set (Seconds)	Training Notes
2	Push-Ups							
		1	To Failure	15+	Bodyweight	1010	60–90	Do as many as you can for each set.
		2	To Failure	15+	Bodyweight	1120	60–90	If you can't do any (or any more), rest for 10–15 seconds then do an initial 1–2 reps or negative reps. This will help advance your strength.
		3	To Failure	10+	Bodyweight	1120	60–90	
		4	To Failure	10+	Bodyweight	1120	45–60	
	Total Reps			50+				
3	Tricep Dips (Body Weight)							
		1	To Failure	10+	N/A	1020	60–90	If you can't do any (or any more), try resting for 10–15 seconds, then doing another 1–2 reps. Also try negative reps, using your legs to push yourself into the straight arm position and lower yourself down.
		2	To Failure	10+	N/A	1020	60–90	
		3	To Failure	10+	N/A	1020		
	Total Reps			30+				
4	Standing (Military) or Seated Shoulder Press							
		1	6	8	70%	1020	90–120	This should be heavy enough that at best you can just lift the optimal target reps, no more.
		2	3	5	80%	1020	90–120	
		3	3	4	80%	1020	90–120	If the weight is right, you should be struggling to lift more than 1 good rep.
		4	2	3	80%	1020	90–120	
		7	8	10	60%	1010	15–30	Drop the weight and pump up the reps.
		8	To Failure	To Failure	45%	1010		You should be struggling to complete more than a few reps.
	Total Reps		22	30				

5 Incline Bench Press (Dumbbells or Barbell)

Set	Reps	%	Tempo	Range	Note
1	6	70%	1020	90–120	*This should be heavy enough that at best you can just lift the optimal target reps, no more.*
2	3	80%	1020	90–120	
3	3	80%	1020	90–120	*If the weight is right, you should be struggling to lift the final rep.*
4	2	80%	1020	90–120	
7	8	60%	1010	15–30	*Drop the weight and pump up the reps.*
8	To Failure	45%	1010		*You should be struggling to complete more than a few reps.*
Total Reps	22	30			

6 Standard Flat Bench Press (2 Weeks Barbell, 1 Week Switch To Dumbbells)

Set	Reps	%	Tempo	Range	Note
1	4	80%	1020	60–90	*This should be heavy enough that at best you can just lift the optimal target reps, no more.*
2	3	80%	1020	60–90	
3	6	70%	1020	45–60	
4	6	65%	1010		*Drop the weight and pump up the reps. You can keep going until failure.*
Total Reps	19	30			

7 Medium (V-Bar or Straight Bar) Grip Triceps (Palms Down/Pronation) Push-Down

Set	Reps	%	Tempo	Range	Note
1	6	75%	1020	60–90	
2	8	70%	1020	45–60	
3	8	50%	1020		*This is a drop set, so you can keep going until failure.*
Total Reps	22	30			

8 Cardio Warm-Down

Set	Time	Note
1	10–15 Min	*Run, bike, skate, whatever you like, just get the blood pumping. You should already be sweating from the training, but don't stop, go fast, go intense, try intervals, finish your workout with pride!*

Note: It's recommended that you include a 3–5 minute low-intensity cool down.

PLATEAU BREAKER PLAN | DAY 3
Time to complete: aim for under 1 hour, max 1 hour 10 minutes (70 minutes)

Day 3

No.	Exercise	Set	Minimum Reps	Optimal Target Reps	Estimated % of One Rep Max	Guide Tempo	Rest Period After Set (Seconds)	Training Notes
1	Cardio Warm-Up							This should start slow (e.g. a light jog), but elevate to around 50–70% of your max effort. Ensure you get the blood flowing, but don't overdo it.
		1	5–10 Min					
Note: You may want to try some static or dynamic stretching. See: Warming Up, Stretching & Cooling Down								
2	Pull-Ups							
		1	To Failure	10+	Bodyweight	1010	60–75	Do as many as you can for each set.
		2	To Failure	10+	Bodyweight	1120	60–90	If you can't do any (or any more), rest for 10-15 seconds then do a further 1–2 reps or negative reps. This will help advance your strength.
		3	To Failure	10+	Bodyweight	1120	60–90	
		4	To Failure	10+	Bodyweight	1120	60–90	
	Total Reps			40+				
3	Assisted Pull-Up Machine							Set the machine to counter at around 30% of your body weight.
		1	To Failure	8+	Bodyweight	1020	60–90	
		2	To Failure	8+	Bodyweight	1020	60–90	Try lowering yourself really slowly and feel the tension in your lats and biceps.
		3	To Failure	8+	Bodyweight	1020	60–90	
	Total Reps			24+				
4	Medium Grip or Wide Grip Lat Pull-Down							
		1	6	8	70%	1020	90–120	This should be heavy enough that you can only just lift 3 reps, no more.
		2	3	4	80%	1020	90–120	
		3	3	4	80%	1020	90–120	
		4	2	3	80%	1020	90–120	If the weight is right, you should be struggling to lift more than 1 good rep.
		5	2	3	80%	1020	90–120	
		6	8	10	60%	1020	15–30	Drop the weight and pump up the reps.

5 Seated Rows (Machine or Cable Machine)

Set	Reps	Reps	%		Rest	Notes
1	6	10	70%	1020	90–120	If the weight is right, you should be struggling to lift the final reps.
2	6	10	70%	1020	90–120	
3	6	8	70%	1020	90–120	
4	6	8	70%	1020	15–30	
5	To Failure	To Failure	50%	1020		You should be struggling to complete more than 5 additional reps.
Total Reps	24	36				

6A Wide Grip (Palms Up/Supination) Ez-Bar Bicep Curl

Set	Reps	Reps	%		Rest	Notes
1	15	20	Bar Only	1010	60-90	Warm Up.
2	3	4	85%	1120	60-90	
3	2	3	85%	1120	60-90	Choose a challenging weight, but make sure you use correct form.
4	2	3	85%	1120	60-90	
Total Reps	22	30				

6B Switch To: Reverse Grip (Palms Down) Ez-Bar Bicep Curl

Set	Reps	Reps	%		Rest	Notes
5	8	10	75%	1020	60-90	Reverse (Pronation) Grip Curls are usually harder than Palms Up (Supination) Curls so you may need to drop the weight. These will also help strengthen your forearms.
6	To Failure	To Failure	50%			
Total Reps	8	10				

7 Cardio Warm-Down

Set	Reps	Notes
1	5–10 Min	Run, bike, skate, whatever you like, just get the blood pumping. You should already be sweating from the training, but don't stop, go fast, go intense, try intervals, finish your workout with pride!

Note: It's recommended that you include a 3–5 minute low-intensity cool down.

APPENDIX

FREE BONUS CONTENT: THELEANEXEC.COM

It's the era of digital! So, rather than load up the appendix with lots of static extra info, as a purchaser of the book you can access a whole range of information, support tools and resources on TheLeanExec.com. I look forward to seeing you there and feel free to get in touch via the contact form on the site if you have any queries.

To access, go to BIT.LY/TLE-BOOK and register or type the link into the address bar on your mobile or PC internet browser.

Book Registration Link:

BIT.LY/TLE-BOOK

Enter your details and the following code:

N8F6LI31QS

IDEAL BODY MEASUREMENT

The concept of ideal body measurements is very subjective and ultimately all bodies have their advantages and disadvantages, even when highly trained. For the purpose of The Lean Exec, the main focus is on ensuring that you have balance and symmetry not only as it tends to look better, but mainly because it's going to give you a more rounded athleticism, strength and fitness.

In male bodybuilding, the classic physique of Steve Reeves was deemed an "ideal" in terms of symmetry and aesthetics. At 6ft 1in (1.854 Meters) and 210lbs (95kg) his stats were:

- ☑ Arms: 18.5 inches
- ☑ Calves: 18.5 inches
- ☑ Neck: 18.5 inches
- ☑ Thighs: 27 inches
- ☑ Chest: 54 inches
- ☑ Waist: 30 inches

If you want more detail on this it's in his book, Building the Classic Physique – The Natural Way or summarized in articles available with a quick search online.

Steve's measurements could be seen as small by comparison to some of the 240 lb+ bodybuilders you see today, but it's still quite big versus the average fit male. For example, it's worth noting that at 1.9 meters (6ft 2in) Chris Hemsworth's appearance as Thor is/was 200lbs (90.7 kg).

Research suggests that even Chris Hemsworth's impressive Thor physique is in the larger size of what most women and men view as "ideal" (and/or appealing). As they say, beauty is in the eye of the beholder and tastes and preferences can vary widely.

Ultimately though, the important thing is, it's all about what you see as ideal, right for you and what you want to achieve, not what other people think. Not to mention that health and fitness should be core to why you exercise and eat well, look should be the added bonus, not essential.

In line with the Symmitarian thinking to achieve balance and realism, we've done some research based on typically what is seen as ideal (and/or considered appealing) to the majority based on height and considering varying body types. If it's of interest, you'd like to explore more and calculate the range for your body, you can access the information and tools here on the site:

BIT.LY/IDEALBODYCAL

BASIC NUTRIENTS

Our bodies need fuel to perform at their best and recover. There are lots of nutrients that are relevant to the body, but some in particular are important to optimising your exercise.

Macronutrients

☑ Protein:

☑ Taken from the definition, protein is nitrogenous organic compounds which have large molecules composed of one or more long chains of amino acids and are an essential part of all living organisms, especially as structural components of body tissues, such as muscle, hair, etc., and as enzymes and antibodies.

☑ Protein is a building block of muscle (tissue) but is an element of all organs within the body and bodily functions. Proteins are formed from 20 amino acids.

Essential Amino Acids:

- Histidine
- Isoleucine
- Leucine
- Valine
- Lysine
- Methionine
- Phenylalanine
- Threonine
- Tryptophan

Non-Essential Amino Acids:

- Alanine
- Arginine

- Asparagine

- Aspartic acid

- Cysteine

- Glutamic acid

- Glutamine

- Glycine

- Proline

- Serine

- Tyrosine

Carbohydrate

☑ Taken from the definition, any of a large group of organic compounds occurring in foods and living tissues and including sugars, starch, and cellulose. They contain hydrogen and oxygen in the same ratio as water (2:1) and typically can be broken down to release energy in the body.

☑ Carbohydrates are the first source of fuel energy for the body. Carbohydrates range from simple, which are more quickly digested and absorbed by the body (e.g. sugar, biscuits, sweets, sugary drinks, etc.) through to complex (e.g. vegetables, beans, grains, etc.) which are digested and absorbed more slowly. The latter are richer in quality and more useful to the body.

Fats

☑ Fats are naturally oily substances occurring in the body under the skin. Fats have higher calories per gram and more energy than the other macronutrients. Fat is a backup energy source to carbohydrates, reserved for when additional energy is required by the body.

Other Basic Nutrients

Water

☑ Water constitutes 60% of the adult male body (55% in adult women) and 72% of the muscle.

For more on recommended water intake, go to:
BIT.LY/TLE-WATER

Micronutrients

☑ Vitamins – any of a group of organic compounds that are essential for normal growth and nutrition and are required in small quantities in the diet because they cannot be synthesised by the body.

☑ Minerals – essential chemicals that assist in vital bodily functions, found in a variety of foods, including some macronutrient foods.

For more on Micronutrients, go to:
BIT.LY/TLE-MICRO

Supplements

☑   Supplements can be used to support a healthy
      diet and ensure your body is getting the appro-
      priate MACRO and MICRO Nutrients it needs to
      support your training.

For more on Supplements, go to:

BIT.LY/TLE-SUPP

THANKS FOR BUYING THE LEAN EXEC BOOK, PUBLISHED BY BIGGER BROTHER LTD.

Sign up and register your book purchase (see appendix for details) to access the free Book support content including alternative exercises and plans, stretching routines, training and nutrition tools, meal planners and more:

BIT.LY/TLE-BOOK

PLEASE REVIEW THE LEAN EXEC BOOK ON AMAZON Reviews mean a lot and are really appreciated, so please take a few minutes to let me know what you thought of this book.

If you haven't already signed up to our exclusive newsletter to access free content, offers and more please visit the link below.

BIT.LY/TLE-SIGN-UP

Once signed up you'll receive regular tips, tricks, hacks, and facts plus exclusive offers and deals for new products and services to help optimise your motivation, health, fitness and results daily.

 #THELEANEXEC

 FACEBOOK.COM/THELEANEXEC

 INSTAGRAM.COM/THELEANEXEC

 THELEANEXEC.TUMBLR.COM

PINTEREST.CO.UK/THELEANEXEC

THELEANEXEC.COM
BIGGERBROTHER.COM